fitness
food

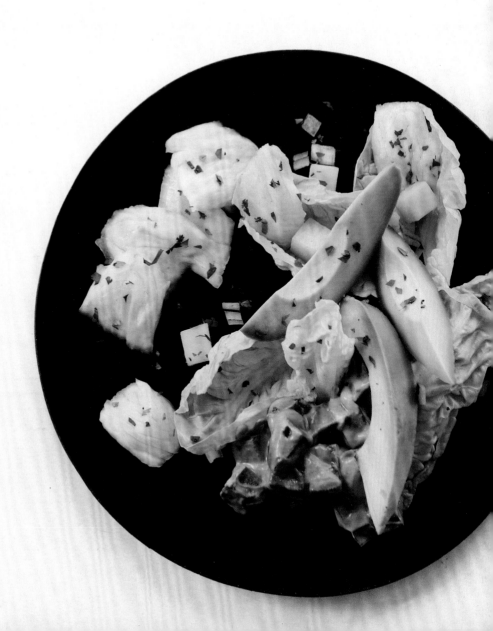

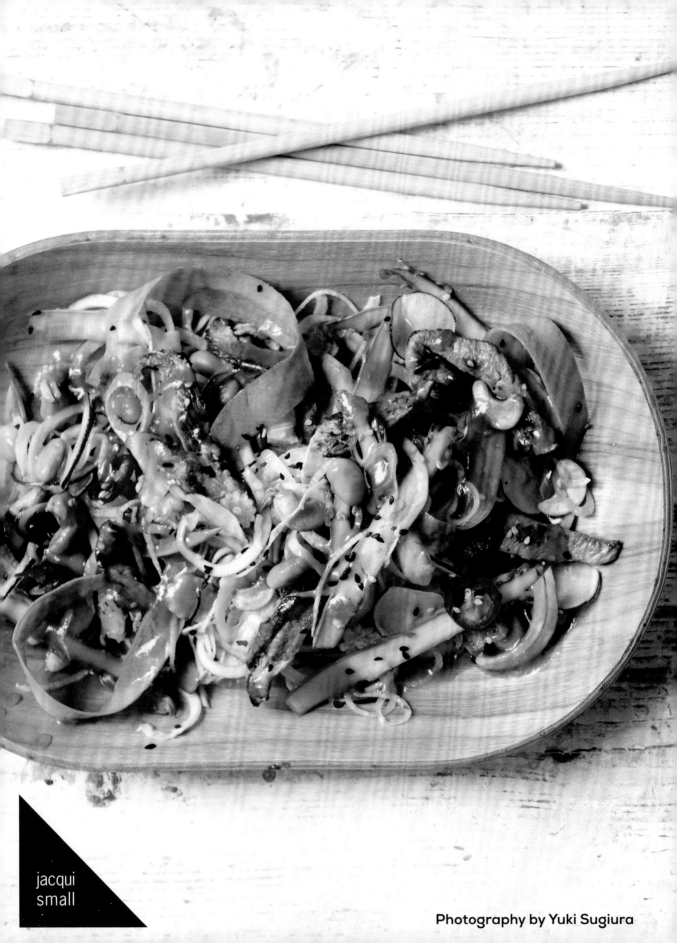

jacqui
small

Photography by Yuki Sugiura

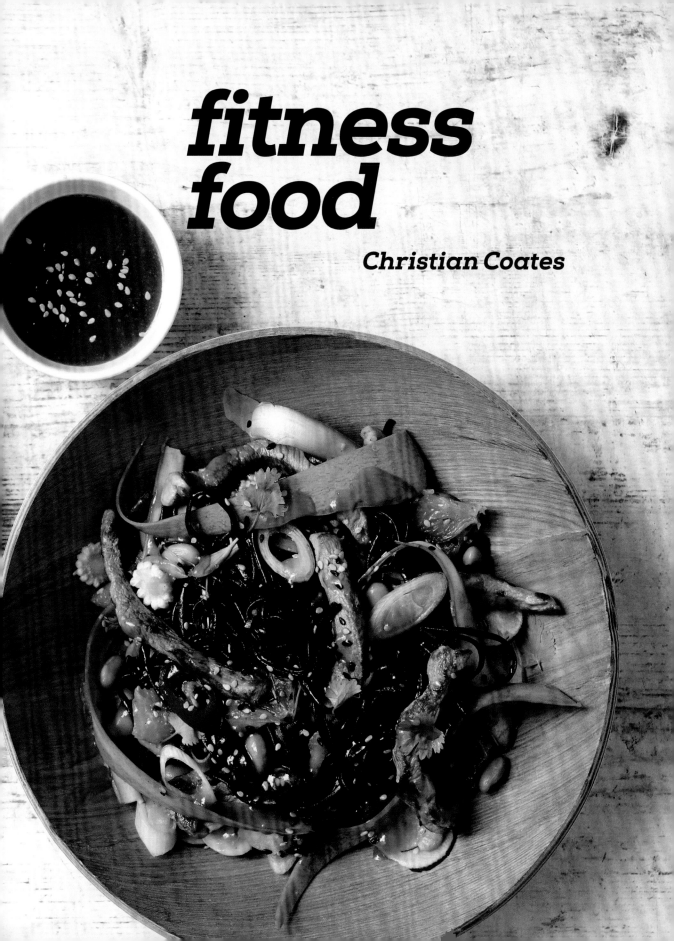

fitness food

Christian Coates

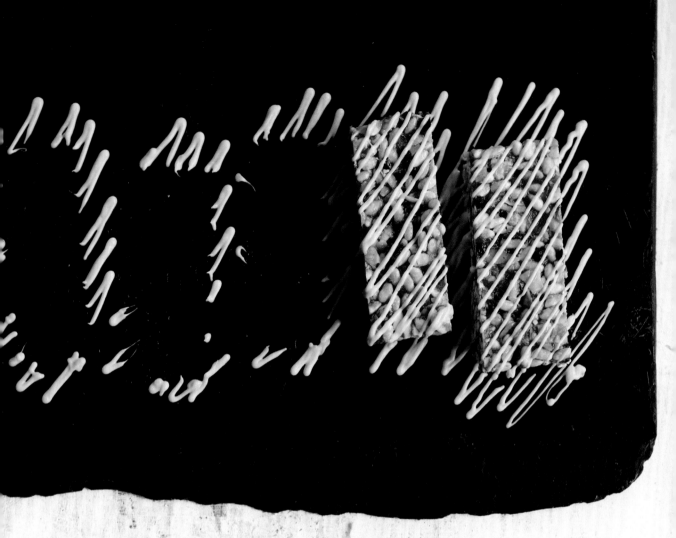

First published in 2015 by
Jacqui Small LLP
74–77 White Lion Street
London N1 9PF

This paperback edition published 2017

Publisher: Jacqui Small
Senior Commissioning Editor: Fritha Saunders
Managing Editor: Emma Heyworth-Dunn
Project Manager and Editor: Nikki Sims
Design and Art Direction: Lawrence Morton
Photographer: Yuki Sugiura
Prop Stylist: Cynthia Inions
Proofreader: Claire Wedderburn-Maxwell
Production: Maeve Healy

ISBN: 978 1 910254 91 2

A catalogue record for this book is available from the British
Library.

2019 2018 2017
10 9 8 7 6 5 4 3 2 1

Printed in China.

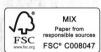

MIX
Paper from
responsible sources
FSC® C008047

Quarto is the authority on a wide range of topics.
Quarto educates, entertains and enriches the lives of
our readers—enthusiasts and lovers of hands-on living.
www.quartoknows.com

Contents

Introduction

Call it a eureka moment, but it suddenly became apparent to me how generic and misleading most off-the-shelf diets are. When people follow set plans from a newspaper or in 'traditional' diet books, they are asked to follow a 'one size fits all' approach. These ineffective plans may start well but they are completely unrealistic and, therefore, unsustainable. Users of such plans often fail as they see results plateauing due to lack of variety or not being able to adapt to fit in with their day-to-day life. Through my own experience, if some days I wasn't able to exercise or I had been travelling, the plan would recommend me to eat certain quantities for that day, regardless of what I was doing. Ultimately, the lack of flexibility meant I would overeat and not get the desired results. Failure was inevitable.

This realisation was the driving force behind the formation of Soulmatefood. I wanted to offer bespoke, tailored nutrition and hassle-free meals direct to the door. Not just strictly aimed at traditional weight loss, but also to fulfil other areas, such as vitality, sports performance, energy and appearance, while utilising top-quality ingredients and vibrant gourmet recipes. Any eating plan needs to be sustainable and this can only be underpinned through education with regard to how and what someone eats – I'm talking portion control, meal frequency, learning which carbs are good, which foods are high in protein, which fats are best and choosing foods that are potent nutritional ingredients.

After working with clients who vary from complete nutritional novices to top-level professional athletes, it became apparent that I needed to design a concept that could deliver a nutritional ethos that worked for all levels. One that could be incredibly simple and basic to follow, or as bespoke (or precise) as you need for specific physical results. Hence *Fitness Gourmet* was born.

The recipes in this book are put together to banish the misconception that healthy food has to be mundane, tasteless and bland. The Soulmatefood team and I are realistic; we aren't the type of people who haven't eaten a carb since the age of 16. We are passionate about flavours, tastes and colours and enjoy creating über-healthy spins on meals that are traditionally seen as indulgent or bad for you. Every dish in this book serves a purpose and this is half the battle, especially getting the carb/protein levels right to fit into each of the three categories! This book has been put together by leading nutritionists and top chefs who we have been fortunate enough to work with. I am delighted to be able to bring such a high level of nutritional knowledge and high standard of recipes into your home.

So, wave goodbye to the days of obsessing about numbers and calorie counting, our ethos is based around portion control, quality of ingredients and ratios of proteins to carbohydrates. The plan is simple to follow and meals can be enjoyed on your own, with a partner (who may have a completely different goal), your family and even the whole office, sports team or group of friends.

I hope you enjoy creating your own specific diet code to stick to, there are plenty of examples in the book to give you inspiration. Not only that, I'm sure you will be motivated to get in the kitchen and start experimenting with ingredients, cooking techniques and tastes and flavours not normally associated with being on a 'diet'.

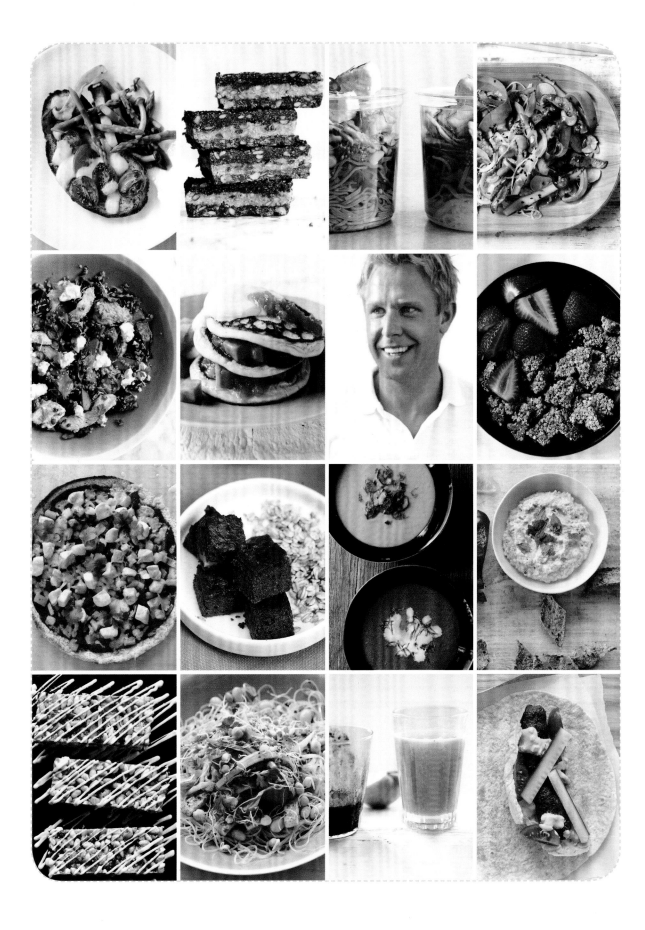

What is the diet code?

The diet code is a simple and straightforward way to achieve your goals for nutrition and fitness. It can be tailored to any goal and any level of fitness and training, from complete beginner to professional athlete. There are three basic levels – Burn, Balance and Build – each with its own symbol.

No decoding needed

The diet code is an at-a-glance way of choosing dishes that do you good, while coordinating with your chosen exercise and level of activity. Every meal has a variation that is shown with the symbols for Burn, Balance and Build. So, if you want to cook, for example, Steak with chicory slaw and salsify chips (see page 183), just look for the relevant symbol on the page and that's the meal you're cooking. With this example, the Balance meal is just as described; the Burn option replaces the salsify chips with celeriac chips; and the Build variation has a steamed corn on the cob as an extra side. It really is that simple.

The easiest and simplest way to reach the goals set out opposite is to follow your chosen symbol for every meal time. Choose this approach if you want simplicity but also great results.

Intermediate and amateur sportspeople can implement a mixed solution: varying their intake by choosing differently coded dishes in line with training or active days. So, for instance, if you know you've got an exercise class on a Tuesday, switch to Build dishes on a Monday to fuel up and get the most out of your active period the next day. Thus, you can customise your menu by the day.

For serious athletes and dedicated sports/gym goers, the concept can be modified by the meal. Maximise performance by fuelling ahead of activities and feeding your body to aid recovery. Switch variations for incredible, tailored results.

Burn 　　　　　*Balance* 　　　　　*Build*

Which diet code is for you?

To discover which variation of the diet code is right for you, look at the lists below and see which tallies most with your goals.

I want to:

▽ lose body fat but maintain lean muscle

▽ burn more fat

▽ reduce health issues associated with excess weight and obesity

▽ tone up.

I want to:

○ maintain current body weight

○ eat a sustainable, healthy diet

○ keep my body in good shape.

I want to:

△ build lean muscle and powers of endurance

△ be able to fuel my body for sport and help it recover

△ increase my body's glycogen storage (energy stores, see page 17).

Other benefits of all the variations include:

→ better regulation of blood sugar levels

→ feeling satisfied when you've eaten (increase satiety)

→ eating foods packed with nutrients

→ increasing energy levels and feeling great

→ boosting powers of focus and concentration.

The ultimate in flexibility

The recipes in this book can be adapted to suit every individual. No more will you have to worry about being on a dreaded 'diet' when you've got friends coming over for dinner. You can still enjoy the same meals with your partner, friends or family by simply modifying certain ingredients; even if they have a completely separate goal, you can still enjoy similar meals together.

As well as changing ingredients for dishes, your code will change as your body starts to change and you feel the benefits after following a diet code for a while. Your diet code is unique to you and your life – there's no 'one size fits all' approach – so the code will differ as you change, as you grow or shrink, as you become more or less active, then the code changes with you and gives you flexibility to stay on track. So, for instance, if you reach your target weight, then switch from the Burn code to the Balance variations of meals; if you've built up enough muscle then switch from Build to Balance or even Burn, if you're looking to reduce body fat.

To see an example of how to mix and match the diet codes with your activity, whether that's football (soccer), pilates or road cycling, take a look at the Eating plans for specific goals (see pages 43–59) that give a visual chart for which type of dishes to eat over the course of a week.

Recipes are for everyone

Dairy has received a bad reputation in the media over the past few years, mainly due to the notion that we are the only species to consume dairy after infancy and also the only species to consume another animal's dairy. It has been suggested that we have not evolved to be able to digest the lactose found in milk as we lose this ability after infancy (when we should no longer require milk, as it is designed to be consumed during the first few years of life) to aid growth and support immunity. However, it appears that only a small percentage of Western Europeans are short of this enzyme, lactose (<10%), and most of us can eat and digest dairy without a problem.

Furthermore, there have been no scientific research papers to suggest any detrimental effects on health of a moderate dairy consumption. Conversely, many papers outline several health benefits. However, if you are lactose intolerant, avoiding dairy products will be at the top of your list of changes to make to your diet. If indeed you are lactose intolerant or chose to follow a dairy-free plan but wish to carry on enjoying the meals in this book, simply swap any dairy ingredients for your favourite non-dairy alternative and make these delicious recipes lactose and dairy free.

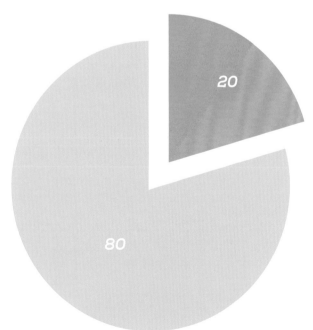

The 80:20 rule

At Soulmatefood we understand the importance of treating yourself now and then, in order to keep on track with your personal goals. Treating yourself or having a 'cheat meal' can be a good tactic to use as you work your way towards a goal. Even though all the Burn meals in this book have been designed with nutritional quality and taste in mind, we appreciate that restricting your choice to one particular variation might feel monotonous. Having a planned 'cheat meal' may help you keep on track by letting you have off-diet-code treats.

As a way of helping you factor in your 'cheat meals', this book has an 80:20 rule, allowing you to enjoy the meals on the Burn diet code 80 per cent of the time; so, treat yourself to a Build or Balance option every now and then, guilt-free! If an option is available as 80:20, it will say so in the variation.

What do the different codes mean?

There are three codes and each one is designed to help you achieve your particular goals. Here's a summary of what each code does and how it does it.

Burn This code is based around restricting carbohydrate intake; but please note this is a 'lower carb' category and not a 'no carb diet'. The general principle for Burn is that when you eat fewer carbs, your body will turn to other sources of energy, such as fat, therefore reducing your body's fat levels.

Balance This code is based around your carbohydrate and protein levels being in equilibrium. Establishing and maintaining a balance of the two can affect the way your body is kept in great shape.

Build By boosting the amount of carbohydrates in your meals, this code fuels your body by increasing energy stores – an essential part of both athletic performance and recovery. This increase in calorie levels, coupled with increased protein intake, also promotes muscle growth and body composition change.

To understand more about the different food types, see Get to grips with the basics, page 14.

You can still enjoy the same meals with your partner, friends or family by simply modifying certain ingredients; even if they have a completely different goal, you can still enjoy similar meals together.

Burn has a protein to carbohydrate ratio of 2:1

Balance has a protein to carbohydrate ratio of 1:1

Build has a protein to carbohydrate ratio of 1:2

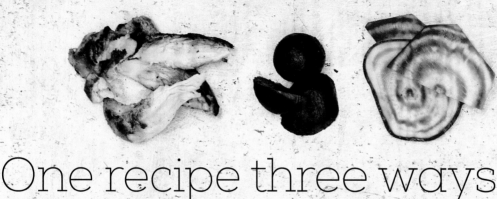

One recipe three ways

It's easy to eat healthily and for ongoing health and happiness with our mouthwatering selection of Soulmatefood's recipes. Don't worry, though, there are no special ingredients or weirdly named foods, all our ingredients are easily sourced, fresh and vibrant.

Eating the Soulmatefood way means you can choose from one of three possible versions of each meal in the book. This ultimate personalisation allows you to opt for Burn if you're trying to shed a few pounds, Build if you're looking to build lean muscle mass or just follow the Balance version for everyday health and vitality. So, you can pick and choose depending on your current goal. What's more, it allows the main cook in a family to cater for several different people with different requirements without cooking three totally different dishes. Great result.

Take one recipe – see how it all works
Here we deconstruct the three variations of the Super-green candy salad with mango and pomegranate (see page 180).

Balance Quinoa is an amazing superfood carbohydrate. Not only is it very low GI (providing a slow-release form of energy), it is also packed full of protein and a full range of amino acids (the building blocks of life), which are usually only found in animal proteins. This nutrient-dense dish contains three servings of fruit and vegetables, providing myriad vitamins, minerals and antioxidants to boost immunity and metabolic function, as well as fighting off free radicals (the highly reactive molecules that cause damage to surrounding molecules and cells).

Burn Remove the quinoa and add leaves. Although quinoa releases its energy slowly, it is still a calorific carbohydrate and so doesn't lend itself well to weight loss and a reduction in body fat. By replacing the quinoa with vibrant green salad leaves, you dramatically reduce calories, while maintaining portion sizes and nutrient density. It won't feel like anything's missing.

Build Add chickpeas and nuts. To add another dimension to this dish and to fuel training or build lean muscle, ramp up your carbs and add chickpeas to boot. Increase the 'good fats' and up the calorie levels by sprinkling cashew nuts or pine nuts over for a wonderfully crunchy topping.

Each recipe has three variations:

Burn Low-fat, very-low-carb and high-protein (follow these variations for weight management and body fat reduction).

Balance Low-fat, low-carb and high-protein (follow these variations for weight management and vitality).

Build High- to moderate-protein and high-carb (follow these variations for packing on lean muscle/ pre- or post-workout and for endurance training).

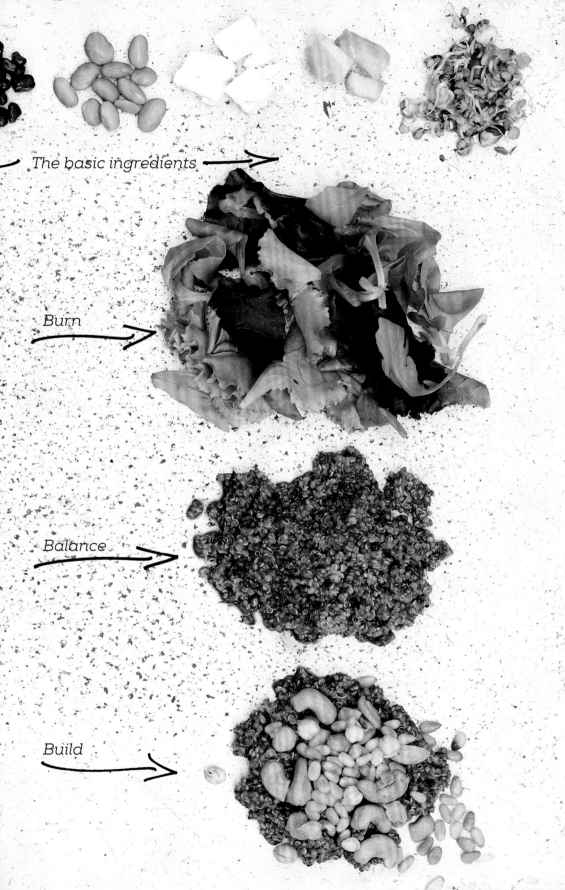

The basic ingredients

Burn

Balance

Build

Get to grips with the basics

If you can understand the basics of nutrition, it's like taking the first step towards changing your nutritional habits for the better.

Nutritional requirements differ from person to person depending on a large array of factors (such as height, weight, metabolic rate, activity level, age and gender), so once you've discovered what the essence of nutrition is (macronutrients and micronutrients, more on this below) you can sit back because Soulmatefood have already done the hard work for you when it comes to planning what to eat.

All the recipes in this book and their variations have been carefully vetted by our nutritional team so that they provide you with all of the components your body needs to be healthy, according to which diet code you're following. So, there's no need to take supplements or make any radical changes in your diet. Now let's find out what it means to eat a healthy, varied and nutritionally sound diet.

Let's talk nutrition

Nutritionists talk of macronutrients and micronutrients, but what exactly are these? When we talk of macronutrients, we are referring to the collective food types of protein, fats, carbohydrates and alcohol (which is included as its own type as it's highly calorific). Micronutrients, on the other hand, are all the minerals and vitamins contained within foods that are important for healthy functioning of your body as well as general maintenance and repair. So, what are these different macronutrients and why are they important for a healthy body?

Protein – building blocks of life

Protein is the second most abundant compound in the body, following water. Protein builds, maintains and repairs your muscles, organs and immune system. The protein you eat in food is broken down into building blocks known as amino acids and then rebuilt as specialised protein molecules wherever and whenever your body needs them. Your body's cells are constantly in a balance of degradation and regeneration, and a readily available supply of amino acids is essential for this process.

What foods provide protein? Sources of protein fall into two categories:

animal-based protein – meats (chicken, turkey, beef, pork, lamb), fish, eggs and dairy produce

plant-based protein – pulses, beans, grains, nuts and seeds.

Proteins are made up of building blocks called amino acids. There are 20 amino acids and our bodies can make 11 of these (the so-called non-essential amino acids) but we have to gain the other nine amino acids (so-called essential amino acids) from the foods we eat.

Animal proteins contain the full spectrum of essential amino acids, whereas plant-based proteins usually contain only a small number of these. So, if you're vegetarian or vegan it's vital that you eat plant-based proteins from a variety of sources to ensure you get the full complement of essential amino acids for health and vitality.

When you eat protein-rich foods you might find you feel fuller for longer. So, eating protein at most meals can help to minimise feelings of hunger.

HOW THE BODY MAKES MUSCLE

Let's talk about muscle growth and repair. Here, the amino acid leucine is king – also known as the 'anabolic trigger'. Leucine is required to kick start the synthesis (production) of proteins. So, when a protein source rich in leucine is eaten a receptor called mTOR (think of it as a gate keeper to muscles that amino acids have to pass through) is activated and allows the amino acids through, thereby increasing protein synthesis. Conversely, if the leucine content of the blood is low the mTOR gate stays well and truly shut. So, as you'll see later on (see Eat to build your body, page 50 or Eat to toughen up, page 53), eating the right type of protein, one that is high in leucine, is key to making muscle proteins.

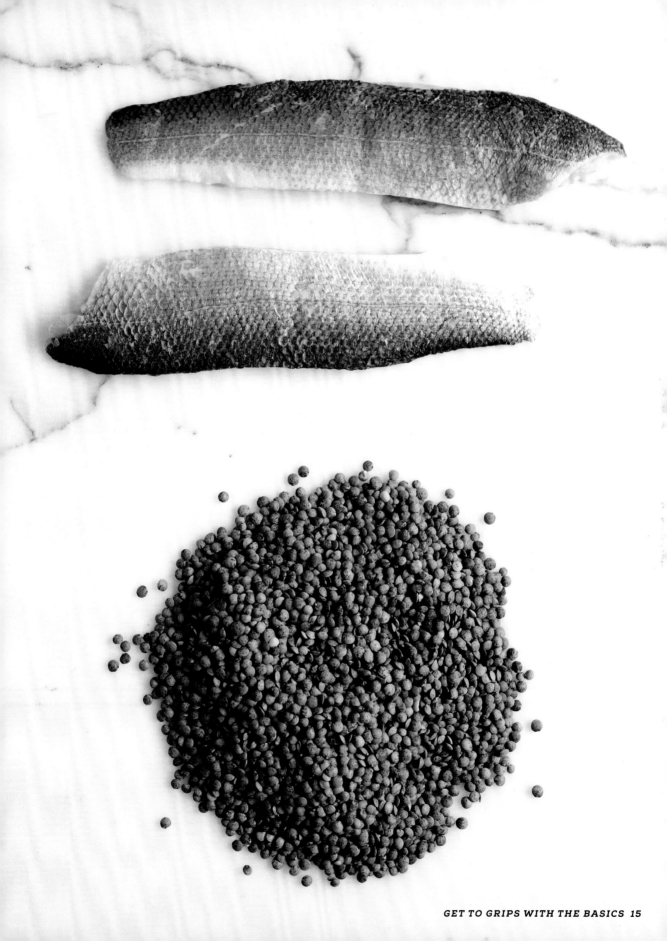

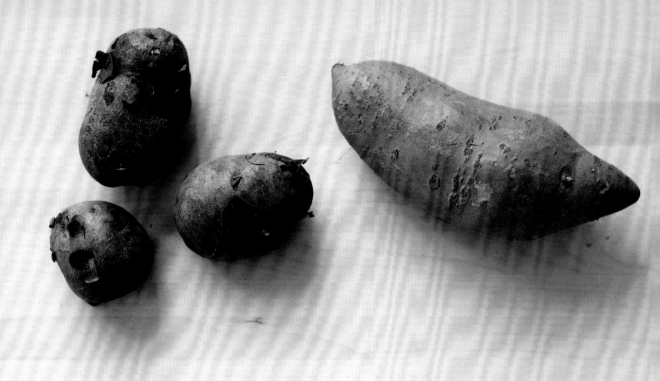

Carbohydrates – friend or foe?

Carbohydrates (or carbs) provide your body with a source of energy. Unlike protein and fat your body does not essentially need carbohydrates but eating them correctly and in moderation can make life easier. Carbs are used as a fuel source during exercise, are the default source of fuel for the brain and are the 'cheapest' form of energy, requiring the least amount of conversion.

What types of foods give you carbohydrates? There are two major types of carbs in foods, known as simple and complex:

simple carbohydrates are sugars, such as glucose (the simplest sugar), fructose (in fruits), sucrose (as refined sugar) and lactose (in dairy produce)

complex carbohydrates, also known as starches, include bananas, barley, beans, breads, cereals, chickpeas, flour, lentils, nuts, oats, pasta, potatoes, root vegetables, sweetcorn and yams. (Where possible, to get the best nutrition, unrefined versions of foods such as cereals, flours and rice should be eaten rather than the refined white versions.)

What is GI? You may well have heard of the term 'GI' with respect to carbs. GI stands for glycaemic index, which is a way of ranking carb-based foods on the overall effect they have on your blood glucose levels. Foods with a low GI mean that they are slowly absorbed in the gut and can release their energy over a longer period of time – they also satisfy you for longer, especially if you choose wholegrain versions. High-GI foods are quickly absorbed and quickly dissipated, leading to big swings in blood sugar, which can leave you reaching for sugary foods and feeling tired and moody. Sugars are high GI, so opt for the lower-GI complex carbs (see also page 39) such as that offered by an oat-based breakfast, for example Spiced honey flapjack breakfast sundae (see page 69) or Strawberry cheesecake yoatie (see page 71).

Many of the carbohydrates in the recipes in this book are low-GI complex carbs, including lots of vegetables and whole grains. Eat carb-dense snacks, such as Lemon cashew bars (see page 112) or Herby edamame dip with buckwheat crackers (see page 107) to fuel exercise or training sessions and also to aid your body's recovery afterwards.

When you eat carbs your body breaks them down into the simple sugar glucose, which is readily used as a fuel source for your brain and also your muscles during exercise.

How your body uses carbs

The process of eating carbohydrates and how they become a fuel source (to be used immediately or stored for later) is complicated. When you eat carbs – whether simple or complex – your body breaks them down into the simple sugar glucose, which is used as a fuel source for your brain and also your muscles during exercise. As sugar levels rise in your bloodstream, a digestive organ called the pancreas releases insulin, which controls the levels of glucose in the blood and allows it to move from the bloodstream into your body's cells.

If you eat a meal that is high in carbs, your blood sugar levels rise rapidly, causing insulin levels to soar, in turn, signalling to cells to take up glucose from the bloodstream to use for energy; if there is plentiful glucose, insulin also prompts your liver and muscles to store glucose in the form of glycogen, after going through a process known as glycogenesis. Conversely, when blood sugar levels are low an enzyme called glucagon releases glucose from glycogen stores in the liver through a process known as glycogenolysis, in turn raising the body's blood sugar levels to a workable level. One thing to note is that muscles do not possess the ability to turn glycogen into glucose except to fuel their own exercise; the glucose freed up for exercise cannot be released into the bloodstream for the rest of the body or even other muscles.

THE FIBRE PROVIDER

Fibre is an essential part of any diet. It comes from the undigestible part of plants and is one of the main reasons for ensuring a good intake of fruit and vegetables in your diet. Fibre as a collective term is made up of two varieties – soluble and insoluble fibre. As you probably can guess, soluble fibre dissolves in water and so tends to reduce the speed of movement of food through the digestive system. Insoluble fibre, on the other hand, does not dissolve in water and so bulks out the food as it makes its way through the intestines. The different fibres have different effects on the body and the food that passes through it.

Soluble fibre can

→ lower LDL (low-density lipoprotein) cholesterol

→ absorb water to form a gel in the stomach, slowing digestion and glucose absorption, helping control blood sugar and insulin levels.

Insoluble fibre can

→ regulate blood sugar

→ promote the movement of food through the intestines, thereby reducing the chance of constipation

→ bulk up stools.

Both forms of fibre can add bulk to a meal without adding calories – you'll feel fuller for longer after a meal and they can therefore help curb overeating.

Fats – essential to life

It's easy to think of fat as bad, but not all fats are equal. Your body needs a certain amount of fat in order to function properly. Every cell in your body has a double layer of fat as an outer membrane and you need an adequate supply of fat in your diet to replenish these and build more cells. Many nerve fibres in your brain and body have a fatty coating to speed nerve signals; fat is vital to a healthy body that can move and respond to its environment.

As well as being an alternative source of energy (fat is, in fact, the richest source of energy, see page 20), fat protects your body's organs, helps you stay warm, helps absorb and transport certain vitamins (A, D, E and K) and helps control chemical reactions around the body.

In the same way that protein is made up of building blocks called amino acids (see page 14), so, too, is fat made from fatty acids. Some of these fatty acids have vital functions in your body but your body can't make them so you have to get them from the food that you eat. These essential fatty acids, as they're known, include omega-3 and omega-6 fatty acids.

So, what makes a fat good or bad? It's not necessarily the amount of fat you eat (though that, of course, does matter) but it's the types of fat that are eaten. Fats can be:

unsaturated (monounsaturated or polyunsaturated) – found in sunflower, rapeseed/canola, olive and vegetable oils and also spreads based on these oils (but not hydrogenated ones), avocados, nuts and seeds and oily fish (mackerel, trout and salmon)

saturated – found in fatty meat and meat products, dairy produce (butter, cheese, cream), pastries, cakes and biscuits/cookies, chocolate, coconut and palm oils.

It's easy to tar all saturated fats with the same brush but, in fact, not all saturated fats are bad. Saturated fats are made up of several different fatty acids that all play different roles within the body. Your body requires a certain amount of saturated fat each day; however, aim to get this from the animal fats and oils as opposed to those in processed foods, such as pastry and biscuits (cookies).

Healthy bodies work better with the majority of dietary fats coming from unsaturated sources, so be sure to include plenty of these in your day-to-day cooking and eating. You'll see later in the recipe section that we use coconut oil in several recipes – and this is a saturated fat. Coconut oil tolerates heat very well, making it perfect for use in frying. Many oils with lower heat tolerances can change the structure of their fatty acids when exposed to high heat, turning them into 'bad' trans-fatty acids. However, this is not the case with coconut oil as the saturated fatty acids are resistant to heat. Another reason why coconut oil should be in everyone's cupboard is that it is beneficial to heart health. Although it is high in saturated fat, the saturated fats found in coconut oil (mainly lauric acid) actually help reduce cholesterol and high blood pressure.

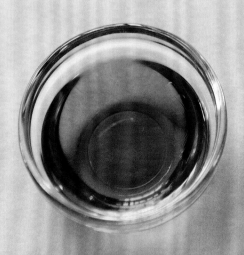

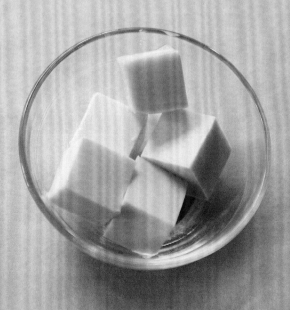

A note on alcohol

As you can see on page 20, alcohol has more calories per gram than protein or carbohydrates. That said, it doesn't have any nutritional value whatsoever. A pint or two a week or a couple of glasses of wine every two weeks isn't going to impact too much on your healthy eating or diet code but as it's so calorific, you do need to be aware of your intake and factor that in.

Your body burns the calories in alcohol first before it starts to burn fat, so if you're following the Burn diet code then drinking alcohol will hinder you achieving your goals.

Drinking a lot of alcohol can impact on how your body responds the following day in terms of how well it recovers from exercise, how it adapts to exercise, your appetite, how you regulate your blood sugar levels and how hard you can train. So, before you head out for a night out, think about not only how it's going to impact on the calorie front but also the havoc it will wreak on your body the next day.

TIPS FOR A LOW-ALCOHOL NIGHT OUT

Trying not to drink alcohol or too much alcohol when surrounded by friends on a night out or when eating out can be hard due to peer pressure. But it's good to limit your intake, your body will thank you: just think of how much closer you will be to achieving your goals. Here are our tips to help limit your intake of alcohol.

→ Have a substantial meal before going out as you will be less likely to want to drink as much if you feel full.
→ Have a 'virgin' version of a cocktail or other alcoholic drink.

→ Opt for spirit-based drinks with low-calorie mixers, as opposed to wine, beers and ciders, as these contain fewer calories and additional substances such as sulphites (which will just add to the head banging the next day) – obviously, that said, drink these in moderation!
→ Alternate a non-alcoholic drink with an alcoholic drink.

PROSECCO
100ml (3½oz) = 74 kcal

GIN AND TONIC
single = 120 kcal
double = 175 kcal

RED WINE
175ml (6oz) = 128 kcal
250ml (9oz) = 170 kcal

WHITE WINE
175ml (6oz) = 129 kcal
250ml (9oz) = 171 kcal

LAGER
½ pint (10oz) = 82 kcal
1 pint (20oz) = 164 kcal

CIDER
½ pint (10oz) = 119 kcal
1 pint (20oz) = 238 kcal

ROSÉ WINE
175ml (6oz) = 133 kcal
250ml (9oz) = 178 kcal

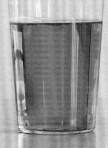
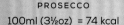
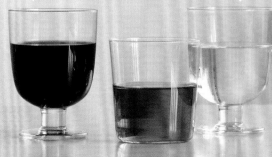

WE ALL NEED ENERGY

As we've learned earlier, we can get energy from various different foods and drinks. Everyone needs energy to fuel their bodies, to grow, be active and keep warm; energy is key for life itself. Different food and drinks provide different amounts of energy; this amount of energy is measured in units of kilocalories (often just referred to as calories) or kilojoules. Here's how the four macronutrients all stack up in terms of energy provision.

Fats 9 kcal per gram

Alcohol 7 kcal per gram

Protein 4 kcal per gram

Carbohydrates 4 kcal per gram

What are micronutrients?

The term micronutrient refers to a broad list of vitamins and minerals. Like the macronutrients, micronutrients are essential for a healthy body, but we only need tiny amounts of these ('micro' is Greek for small). Vitamins and minerals play a crucial role in healthy growth and development, are crucial cofactors in metabolism and energy balance and play a crucial role in the regulation and activation of other micronutrients. If you're lacking a particular mineral or vitamin, you could end up feeling tired, unable to concentrate or always unwell.

We like to think of micronutrients as the cement between the macronutrient building blocks; a wall can be built of the biggest bricks but it easily falls down without the cement holding the bricks together, the same goes for your body. You might look 'ripped' and 'built' on the outside but the inside of your body could be a mess if you have neglected certain vitamins and minerals.

Minerals include calcium, iron, magnesium, potassium, sodium and zinc.

Vitamins most take letters and sometimes letters and numbers, including A, B, C, D, E and K.

If you eat a varied diet, you should easily consume your recommended intake of vitamins and minerals. If your diet is too narrow, you could easily become deficient and need to consult a nutritionist.

How the body makes energy

Different people need different amounts of energy – it depends on your basal metabolic rate (BMR), which measures the amount of energy your body uses to maintain basic functions, such as breathing and heart beating, but it doesn't take into account any activity, even basic activity. Everyone's BMR is different due to it being affected by many factors: height, weight, age, gender, muscle mass and body fat. But when it comes to guidelines on calorie consumption, recommendations are generalised and state that men should aim to eat a total of 2500 kcal a day and women 2000 kcal. However, such figures are likely to be incorrect for most people's requirements, so should be viewed with caution.

As you'd expect some activities use more energy than others. The more active you are, the more energy your body uses up. For example, if one day your daily exercise regime burns 450 kcal, you walk to work (burning 150 kcal) and burn a further 300 kcal from moving around during the day, you will be adding an extra 900 kcal to your energy expenditure on top of what is needed to match your BMR. Being physically active can also increase your muscle mass and this means you will actually be using more energy all the time, even when you are sitting on the sofa. People with similar weight but higher body fat percentage will more than likely have a lower BMR than those with a lower body fat percentage (and therefore higher muscle mass) as muscle has a higher metabolic activity level than fat.

Jargon busting – the science made simple

Throughout this book you may come across some scientific terms that you may not have heard of previously. But here's our go-to page for any terms where you'd like to know more.

BMD – Short for bone mineral density; the lower a person's BMD the higher their risk of bone-related health issues.

Cardiac output – This is the volume of blood pumped out of the heart in 1 minute.

Electrolytes – These mineral salts are very important for the efficient functioning of the brain, nerves, heart and muscles as these minerals carry electrical signals across membranes. The different electrolytes (sodium, potassium, calcium and magnesium) all play different roles in the body.

Energy balance – How many calories you consume versus how many you burn. A positive energy balance is one where you are eating more calories than you are burning; a negative energy balance is when you are eating fewer calories than you are burning.

GI – Shorthand for glycaemic index, GI is a measure of how quickly a given ingredient increases blood glucose levels; the index runs from 0 to 100, so low-GI ratings are at the lower end of numbers and high-GI ratings are up nearer 100. Many people talk about GI (see also page 16), but we think the more relative and useful indicator of blood sugar control is glycaemic load (GL).

GI distress – Gastrointestinal distress, to give its full name, is a long term for a stomach upset. It's a feeling of sickness after eating a certain food or too much of a certain food.

GL – Glycaemic load measures the effect of the glycaemic index of the carbohydrate content of the meal, so it is a much more relevant measure than GI when planning meals. For example, let's take watermelon, which has a high GI value of 72. But as watermelon contains only 5g of carbohydrate per 100g, the GL is only 3.6 for a 100g (3½oz) serving, which would be lower than the equivalent size serving of brown rice.

Glycogen – After eating a carb-based meal, there will more than likely be excess glucose that the body does not need for energy. This excess is stored in the muscles and liver as glycogen (think of it as an energy bank, so it is saved for another time). The average adult can store around 500g (1lb 2oz) of glycogen, providing enough energy for 90 minutes of running or endurance activity; after this time you'll need extra glucose in the form of bananas, energy gels and other high-carb snacks.

HDL cholesterol – Also known as the 'good' cholesterol, this high-density lipoprotein maintains blood vessel health by cleaning and removing LDL cholesterol and transporting it to the liver for recycling.

Hydration status – Technical term for whether you are hydrated or not (see page 22).

Insulin – The hormone responsible for reducing blood sugar levels by allowing cells to take up glucose for energy, causing muscles and liver to store glucose as glycogen and for fat cells to uptake fat.

LDL cholesterol – Also known as the 'bad' cholesterol, this low-density lipoprotein cholesterol contributes to increased risks of heart attacks and strokes. The LDLs collect on the walls of blood vessels, increasing the chances of blockages and clots forming due to these obstructions.

Osteopenia – A lower than normal bone mineral density (see BMD above) that is not low enough to be classed as osteoporosis; it's like a warning sign that bone strength needs to be improved or osteoporosis may occur. This condition is most frequent in post-menopausal women (due to lower oestrogen levels), anyone with a poor diet, female athletes, certain groups of male athletes and those who rarely perform any weight-bearing exercises.

Osteoporosis – A progression of osteopenia, which occurs from further decreased BMD if no action is taken. If a person has osteoporosis the bones are much more fragile, which increases the risk of fractures.

Power to weight ratio – This is a performance factor of many sports and basically shows how powerful you are for your weight – so a lighter person who is as powerful as a heavier person will have a higher power:weight ratio.

Protein synthesis – The process of making new protein (muscle), see also page 14.

Stroke volume – The volume of blood pumped from the left ventricle of the heart in a single contraction, measured in millilitres/beat.

What does water do for you?

All living things need water to survive. Without water, your body would stop working properly. Water makes up about 60-65 per cent of your body weight (depending mostly on how much body fat a person has: more body fat less water, less body fat more water), and a person can't survive for more than a few days without it. Your body uses water for many important normal functions: regulating body temperature, acting like a shock absorber for joints and body organs, transporting nutrients to and through cells, keeping mucous membranes moist and flushing out waste products.

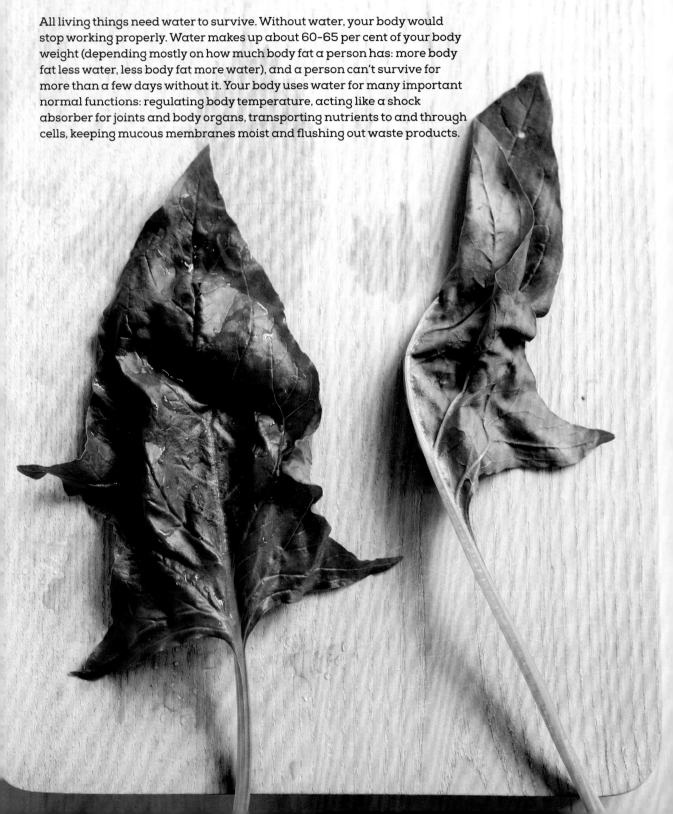

How you lose fluid

On average, a person sweats about 500ml (18oz) each day, but that's before you take into account the temperature of the environment or frequency of exercise or activity (see Factors affecting fluid loss below). In addition to this volume of sweat, we lose almost 250ml (9oz) of water daily just through breathing. Every time we breathe out (exhale) our breath contains water in the form of water vapour. Within this water vapour are electrolytes (minerals such as sodium and potassium, see page 21), so we'll be losing a quantity of these too.

It's important to be aware of how easily you can become dehydrated if you are not actively replacing any lost fluids. What's more, you do not have to be exercising or in the heat to dehydrate, you can dehydrate simply sitting at a desk in a cold office if your fluid intake does not match your fluid losses.

For healthy body function, you need to replace these losses throughout the day every day – and you do this through the food you eat and the drinks you consume (see pages 24–25).

WHAT WATER DOES FOR YOUR BODY

→ moistens mucous membranes in your mouth, eyes and nose

→ regulates body temperature

→ lubricates joints

→ protects body organs and tissues

→ helps prevent constipation

→ reduces the burden on kidneys and liver by flushing out waste products

→ helps dissolve water-soluble minerals and other nutrients (including vitamins B complex and C) to make them accessible to the body

→ helps carry nutrients and oxygen to all cells.

SIGNS OF DEHYDRATION

If you spot any of the giveaway signs of dehydration below, make sure you increase your fluid intake to counter the dehydration:

→ tiredness

→ headache and/or nausea

→ feeling too hot

→ a dry mouth or cough

→ flushed skin

→ a loss of appetite

→ light-headedness

→ dark and strong-smelling urine.

FACTORS AFFECTING FLUID LOSS

Now you know what hydration is, you need to understand what can make you dehydrated so then you can become more aware of potential fluid loss. Once you are aware of all the factors that affect fluid losses you will be able to actively combat these by proactively increasing your fluid intake.

Temperature The temperature of the environment you are in can play a significant role in how much fluid you lose through sweating. The higher the temperature, the more you sweat as your body strives to maintain its core temperature.

Wind speed When outside – whether training, playing sport or casually walking – wind speed can impact on sweating rates. If it's windy, the sweat you produce will evaporate quickly, cooling you down more efficiently; at lower wind speeds, you sweat more as it doesn't evaporate so fast.

Humidity When the environment's humidity is high, you sweat more and continually, as there's no scope for your sweat to evaporate to cool you down; the opposite stands for lower humidity situations, where you sweat much less as your sweat cools you efficiently as it evaporates.

Training intensity The harder you work and move about, the more heat is generated by your body, which increases your body temperature and so you sweat more.

Non-breathable clothing Clothing will affect your sweat rate in a similar way to humidity. If your clothing is non-breathable, the humidity at your skin's surface will increase, reducing evaporation and, therefore, reducing cooling.

Drink little and often

When nutritionists talk about hydration or hydration status, what they mean is the balance of water in the body as a whole, right down to a cellular level. It's not simply a reflection of how much water you've drunk. To be hydrated, all your body's cells have to receive fluids and use them effectively.

To stay hydrated throughout the day, it is important to drink moderate amounts frequently – so find a drink you like the flavour of (not caffeinated, sugary or fizzy drinks, obviously). Drinking 2 litres (8 cups) in an hour as you're suddenly feeling parched might almost match the recommended volume of water to drink in a day but it won't leave you hydrated, as much of this liquid will pass straight through you, without being absorbed by the gut into the bloodstream, and therefore not entering any of your body's cells.

So, the mantra is drink before you're thirsty – moderate amounts throughout the day.

Minimising dehydration for sport

It can be difficult to drink enough fluids to stay hydrated while you're exercising or training, therefore the aim instead is to minimise dehydration. If your body becomes dehydrated past a certain level (2 per cent of your body weight), it can have detrimental effects both on your health and on your performance, especially during any endurance events.

How does dehydration affect performance? As dehydration occurs, fluid levels in the blood drop, causing the blood's viscosity (or its thickness) to rise and blood volume to fall, this in turn causes the heart rate to increase. As the heart rate rises, the volume of blood pumped out of the heart with each heartbeat (known as the stroke volume) is reduced, due to the shorter amount of time the heart has to fill with blood. In addition to these effects on the body's cardiovascular system, dehydration also increases your body's core temperature, increases glycogen utilisation (see pages 17 and 21) and decreases central nervous system function, which translates physically as losses of focus, concentration and coordination.

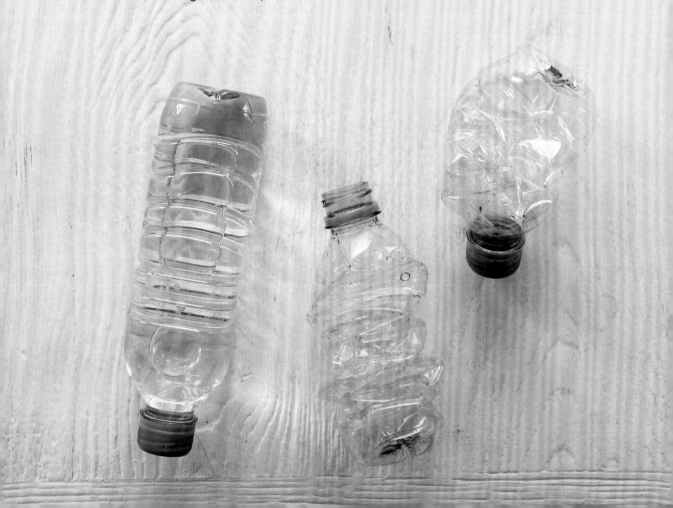

It is vitally important to ensure that you start any training or competition fully hydrated. So, 2–3 hours beforehand be sure to drink 500ml (2 cups) of water with electrolytes (always drink electrolytes when doing any exercise, see below). If your urine is not a pale yellow before you start your activity, be sure to drink a further 250ml/1 cup (of water with electrolytes) 1 hour beforehand.

What are electrolytes?

Electrolytes are essential minerals that allow your body to function well. During exercise, increased amounts of electrolytes are lost during sweating, and these need to be replaced. The electrolyte sodium is required for the absorption of water through the small intestine; if you drink plain water without sodium after exercise a large percentage of the liquid will go straight through the small intestine without being absorbed, thereby having no effect on your hydration. The electrolytes calcium, magnesium and potassium also need replacing in fluids as they play roles in muscular contraction and the function of the heart, brain and nervous system.

CALCULATING FLUID LOSSES

A simple and easy yet effective way to ensure you are properly rehydrating is to keep track of your weight before and after training. Weight loss during training is predominantly water loss (with some muscle glycogen loss and even less fat loss).

Weigh yourself before and after training; any weight you have lost will be fluid and so needs to be replaced. As a rule of thumb, try to drink 1.5 times the weight you have lost. So, for instance, if you've lost 0.5kg (1.1lb) then drink 0.75 litres (3¼ cups) to counteract that fluid loss.

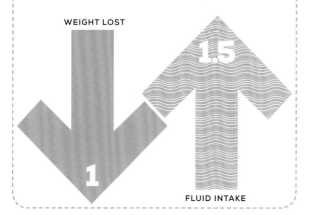

WEIGHT LOST

FLUID INTAKE

Top drinks for good hydration

How much should you drink? As we mentioned above, your body gets water not just from drinks but also from the food you eat. In percentage terms, you should get about 20–30 per cent from food and 70–80 per cent from drinks, preferably water. That said, current advice recommends that men should drink 2.5 litres (10½ cups) on a daily basis and women 2 litres (8 cups) a day.

Drinking only water may not be the most effective way to maintain hydration or rehydrate, as we learned earlier. The advantages of electrolytes in sports drinks are well known due to the huge marketing budgets of these companies; however, these drinks are often also full of sugars, sweeteners and colourings. You will be glad to know there are natural alternatives, with great electrolyte profiles, out there that can also keep you well hydrated (see our Top 5 drinks below). Combining the electrolytes found in fruits and vegetables with water can help aid hydration as opposed to drinking pure water.

Here are Soulmatefood's Top 5 naturally hydrating drinks, all of which provide you with hydration and a good serving of vitamins and minerals – bonus!

1. Coconut water – this drink is currently receiving a lot of attention for its hydrating properties; we can't get enough of it at Soulmatefood.

2. Reset – apple, cucumber and kiwi smoothie (see page 231).

3. A proconut shake – choose any flavour you like (see page 226).

4. Radiance – avocado, pineapple, mint, lime and apple juice (see page 235).

5. Boost – a delicious peanut, banana, nutmeg and honey shake (see page 236) for those looking to aid post-exercise recovery; this is a high-calorie shake.

Grazing is good

Frequent eating – aka grazing – is one of those health topics that comes around on a media press cycle – one year it's good to graze and the next it's to be avoided at all costs. At Soulmatefood, we think grazing is a great way to control what you eat whether your goal is to drop, maintain or gain weight – and that's why we think you should eat a mid-morning and a mid-afternoon snack. As we see it, grazing can have varied effects on your body, which can help you to achieve your goals.

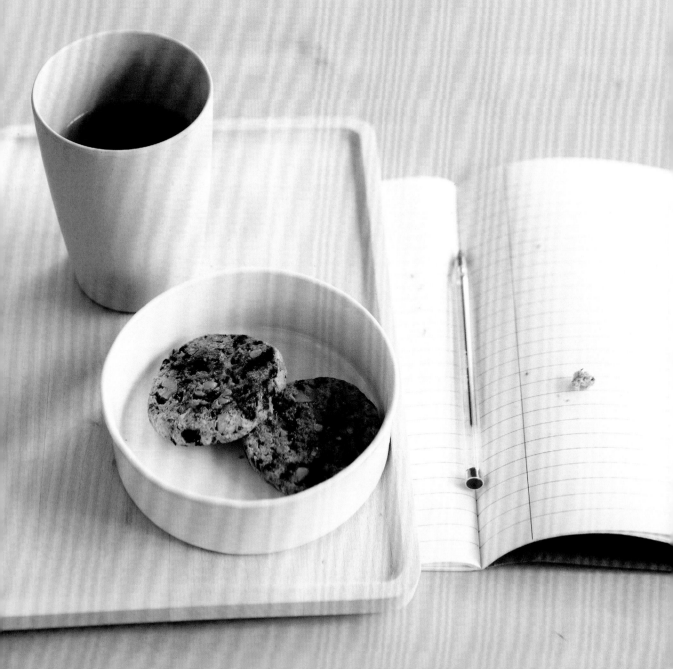

Burn

For those of you following the Burn diet code, you are aiming to lose body fat not body weight. When trying to lose body fat, grazing can help maintain lean muscle mass (which can also maintain metabolism). Graze on protein-based foods every 3–4 hours – as you'll see most of our recipes are protein based. When combined with resistance or weight training, grazing can maximise the manufacture of muscle proteins, and as a result help maintain lean muscle. Lean muscle is a lot more metabolically active than the equivalent amount of fat, for instance, so preserving the muscle may help you burn more calories when compared with losing an increased amount of muscle mass.

Research carried out among professional boxers showed that those who ate six times per day lost the same amount of body weight, but maintained more muscle than those who consumed all their calories for the day at two sittings. This would suggest that frequent eating can help maintain as much lean muscle as possible, which will help you maintain your metabolism, in turn burning more calories and increasing the rate of body fat loss – which is the result you want. Grazing also helps improve your power to weight ratio (one of the most important performance indicators in sport; see page 21) as you reduce weight.

When you eat, the food you've eaten has to be broken down into its constituent parts by your body (the chewing, swallowing, churning and processing in the gut) and this all requires a certain amount of energy – this is known as the thermic effect of food. Many people believe that eating frequently increases metabolism, due to misunderstanding this thermic effect. The idea that grazing directly boosts metabolism is not supported by clinical research, which has mixed findings as to whether frequent meals increase the amount of energy used to digest the food. Some research findings show that eating frequently initiates more frequent, smaller, shorter increases in metabolism, whereas eating larger meals less often would initiate a larger and longer increase in metabolism. In the long run both totalled the same amount of calories burned. Other research supports the findings from this study, so it appears that in reality grazing does not increase metabolism.

So, while grazing does not directly increase metabolism, snacking between meals can help maintain lean muscle, which in turn helps with your weight-loss goals by burning more calories so you lose body fat not just body weight.

Balance

As we've mentioned before, insulin is a hormone that's released to help maintain blood sugar levels and get it into cells, where it's turned into glycogen or stored as fat to be used later for energy (see also page 17). And many of you will be familiar with the sugar highs and lows that mimic the action of insulin as it's released in response to carbohydrate-rich foods, with a higher release associated with more sugary foods. Insulin is also released in response to protein intake. Some research has shown that the insulin response is another element that can be improved with smaller, more frequent meals: results showed lower glucose and insulin levels in the blood when four smaller meals were eaten compared with one large meal containing the same amount of food and total calories. Another study concluded that insulin was reduced by just over 25 per cent when the participants consumed 17 snacks per day as opposed to three meals a day. Obviously, eating 17 snacks per day is a little extreme but what this research helps show is that an increase in meal frequency may help reduce insulin's response.

Other clinical research has shown that a group of people who ate six times per day had lower LDL cholesterol levels (see page 21); these were 5 per cent lower than those of people eating twice a day. Much research backs this up: increased meal frequency results in lower LDL cholesterol concentrations.

Grazing has also been shown to help you take control over your appetite as well as decreasing hunger, as long as the meals are of a good composition. When we say grazing, we don't mean snacking on high-sugar, processed or high-fat foods, such as crisps (potato chips) or sweets (candies); all foods should be the best quality you can afford and always serving a nutritional purpose – real food not adulterated food.

So, snacking between main meals while looking to maintain weight may have a beneficial effect upon several body functions, including reducing 'bad' cholesterol, reducing insulin levels and improving control over appetite; all of which can help you keep a balanced weight.

All of the above grazing benefits can also be applied to the Burn and Build diet codes.

Build

For those of you following the Build diet code, all of what's gone before stands for you too. As mentioned, eating protein-based foods every 3–4 hours helps to maximise protein synthesis – build muscle. When muscle building is your main goal, eating more calories alongside eating more often will help support maximal muscle growth.

But it's not just a case of eating as often as you like; if only. Research suggests that it is possible to eat too often if you're focused solely on gaining muscle mass. Eating high-protein foods means your body is exposed to high levels of amino acids (the building blocks of protein, see also page 14). But muscle appears to reduce in its sensitivity to these amino acids if exposed for a long period of time. When muscles are exposed to high levels of amino acids every 3–4 hours (as we suggest on the Build code), muscle protein synthesis is increased. However, one study showed that when amino acids were provided at 70 per cent above normal levels for several hours the synthesis of muscle protein started to return to normal rates even though amino acid levels remained high. Other research has shown that having a peak in supply of amino acids followed by a drop off to baseline levels allows the body to make greater amounts of muscle protein compared with maintaining high amino acid levels. This suggests that eating protein more often than every 3–4 hours may, in fact, be detrimental to muscle gains. So, don't be tempted to eat much more often as you won't feel any real benefit and it may actually reverse some of the good you've done already.

Many people who are looking to gain muscle need to eat more calories. Grazing can help with that – for instance, it's much easier to eat six 500 kcal meals than three 1000 kcal meals if you're trying to consume 3000 kcal a day. So, eating protein frequently (every 3–4 hours) will help maximise protein synthesis and make it easier to cram in additional calories, leading to increased muscle building capabilities. However, eating more often than this may reduce how much muscle you can build, so try to stick to the guidelines we set out.

Your route through the day

While planning your day's food intake try to give each meal a specific purpose, and don't look at food as 'just food'. Attaching a function to every ingredient and meal that you eat will make you actively think more about your meals and why you are planning, preparing and eating it – you'll find such benefits noted at the top of every recipe later in the book. In this section we will attach a purpose to each meal, depending on whether your goal is Burn, Balance or Build. Aim to eat these meals at intervals of 3-4 hours, so your day looks something similar to this example.

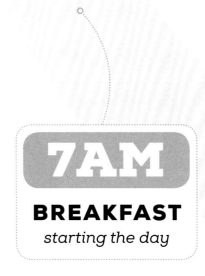

7AM

BREAKFAST
starting the day

Literally coming from 'breaking the fast' of overnight, the first meal of the day is one of the most important. Whatever your goal, breakfast is the perfect time to have a hit of protein and kickstart protein synthesis, as during the night there will have been a significant drop. You want to start protein synthesis early in the morning as your body will have been breaking down muscle overnight, as you haven't eaten for 8–12 hours. Having protein at breakfast will help stop the breakdown of muscle and, if looking to build muscle, will start the building process again.

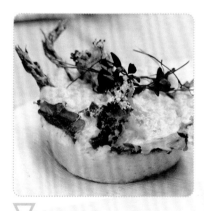

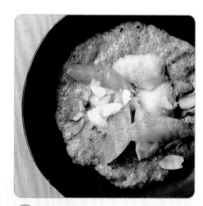

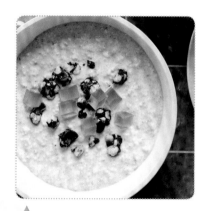

Burn During the night, your blood sugar levels will have dropped and your body concentrates its efforts on metabolising fat. To prolong this increase in fat metabolism, breakfasts need to have a minimal carbohydrate component to keep your blood sugar levels low and fat breakdown high. But foregoing carbohydrates doesn't mean losing out on great taste or nutrition: choose from Coconut pancakes with papaya and macadamia butter (see page 81) or scale down Buckwheat and maple crispies with strawberries (see page 66) or Broccoli, Peppadew and feta mini frittatas with asparagus (see page 96) for a super-fast but delicious meal on the go.

Balance Eating a balanced, low-GI carbohydrate meal first thing in the morning will help set you up for the day. What's more, it reduces the chance of a peak in blood sugar and helps reduce the mid-morning crash that can often be seen after eating high-GI, low-protein commercially produced breakfast cereals. Why not try a new kind of porridge (oatmeal)? The Semolina and chia porridge with orange, lemon and ginger (see page 79) totally fits the bill. Otherwise, opt for American pancakes, your way (see page 83) or make a batch of Coco choc crunch (see page 66) so you've got a breakfast handy if time is tight.

Build To fuel your training for the day, choose a high-carb, low-GI breakfast to increase glycogen stores. Upping the carb content at breakfast will promote a combination of boosting the amount of amino acids being forced into the muscles by insulin and an increased calorie intake, aiding recovery and increasing muscle growth when coupled with resistance training. The yoaties, such as 'After Eight' yoatie (see page 72), are great go-to breakfasts for those following the Build code, but Banana and walnut bread with Earl Grey cream (see page 97) is also a quick breakfast option. If you fancy something more filling at the weekend or when you have more time, then go for the Healthy English breakfast (see page 86).

Top tip If you need an energy boost while you're following this low-carb diet code, simply add a teaspoon of coconut oil to your morning cuppa; it will help to maintain lean muscle, too. The type of fat known as medium-chain triglycerides found in coconut oil are rapidly absorbed by the body, thereby providing an easy-to-use energy source, helping you steer clear of sugary carbs.

Top tip Add a serving of greens powder (such as spirulina) to your morning glass of juice or water for a super-boost of vitamins and minerals. This supplement shouldn't be a substitute for plenty of fruit and vegetables in your normal diet.

Top tip If you're trying to increase your calorie intake, then partner your breakfast with one of the smoothies – Radiance (see page 235) is a refreshing combo of avocado, pineapple, lime, mint and apple; or for something more comforting try a proconut smoothie (see page 226).

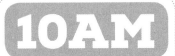

10AM

MID-MORNING SNACK

powering through till lunch

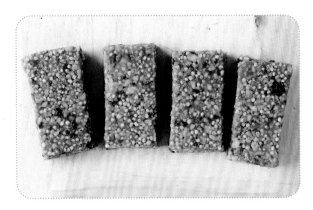

Use this mid-morning snack to help curb your hunger until lunchtime while also giving your body another hit of protein.

Balance A high-protein, low-carbohydrate snack, such as Lemon cashew bars (see page 112) or Vietnamese paper rolls with a fragrant sauce (see page 139) can help reduce hunger to keep you trooping on until lunch, while helping to retain that hard-earned muscle mass.

Snacks are great for refuelling and helping your body recover after exercise. If, for instance, you've had a moderately intensive activity session, then choose from the Balance coded snacks; if you've had a hard training session, then opt for one of the Build coded snacks. Burn snacks are great for less active days.

Top tip After training aim for 20-30g protein and 20-30g carbohydrate for moderate intensity or 40-60g for higher-intensity training; in simpler terms, if you had an easy session then choose a Balance snack and if you've worked hard then have a Build snack.

DRINK THROUGHOUT THE DAY

Hydration goes hand in hand with eating in terms of making reaching your goal that bit easier (see also pages 22–25). A simple approach is to drink a glass of water with every snack and meal and one glass of water between meals, plus at least 500ml (2 cups) per hour when exercising (with added electrolytes to boost absorption of this fluid).

It is good to know that a moderate intake of coffee has been shown not to affect hydration any less than water, so you're free to enjoy a ritual cup in the morning, but for the rest of the day try to stick to water, herbal teas and fruit teas.

Fruit juices, although they contribute to fluid intake, are full of sugar, albeit 'naturally occurring' sugar; the fructose found in fruit should be limited. If you like to drink fruit juice, enjoy it alongside a main meal to lessen the sugar's effects on insulin production and stick to a maximum of one glass per day.

LUNCH
meeting the day head on

Most often, lunches are during a working day, so some preparation is needed for a healthy and nutritious lunch that fits with your diet code.

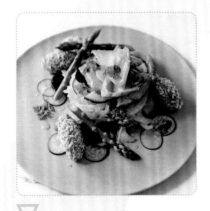

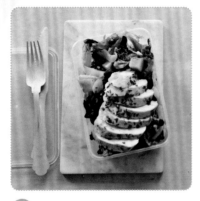

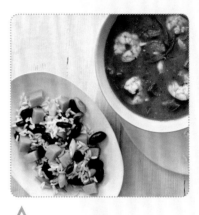

▽

Burn Lunch is an ideal time to treat yourself to a small portion of low-GI carbohydrate – such as Smoked salmon with goat's cheese salad (see page 210). If you like a lighter lunch option, choose a soup such as Super-green pearl barley soup (see page 144). The carbs in lunch will help fuel your brain so that you can concentrate on the tasks at hand during the afternoon shift, helping you work well all the way through to home time! As you are likely to be active in the afternoon – be it getting home from work, walking around at work, cooking in the evening, anything other than sitting still – this serving of carbs will likely be used as an energy source as opposed to being stored as fat.

○

Balance As you are looking to maintain weight and can afford a few extra calories here and there, it may be tempting to reach for an easily accessible but not-so-healthy supermarket or fast-food option. While you may not gain weight with such an approach, you may well experience an 'afternoon crash' at around 3–4pm. So, with the Balance code, opt for a low-GI, balanced carb intake packed full of veggies, which will help control insulin levels and help you stay alert and ready to work while nearby colleagues drift off. Chicken with giant couscous, fennel, pear and walnuts (see page 152) and Halloumi, salsa verde and pasta salad (see page 214) are good options.

△

Build Lunchtime offers you a guilt-free opportunity to cram in the carbs. If you have trained in the morning, the meal's purpose will be recovery; if you're training later in the day then lunch becomes more of a fuelling meal. Either way the fundamentals of the meal are the same – a high-carb and high-protein composition; choose from something like Chilli chicken ramen (see page 159) or Creole gumbo with red beans and rice (see page 194).

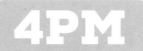

4PM

MID-AFTERNOON SNACK

powering through till dinner

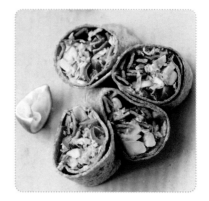

See this snack like the mid-morning snack: as a great way to keep you alert through the afternoon, reducing hunger pangs and allowing you to fully focus on the job at hand. If you're training in the afternoon, eat a Build snack 1 hour beforehand to aid recovery afterwards.

Top tip To boost your mid-afternoon pick-me-up, partner your snack with a cup of green tea. It not only provides a hit of caffeine but is also packed full of antioxidants and phenolic compounds. Another exciting ingredient that gives green tea the upper hand over coffee is that it contains L-theanine, which when consumed with caffeine has a synergistic effect on improving brain function. Bonus!

ADJUST TO SUIT YOUR OWN TIMETABLE

The meal timings shown on this route through your day are only examples and can be adapted to suit your daily routine. Don't feel you have to follow the exact times of what we've suggested here but do try to stick to the 'a meal every 3 hours' format to take advantage of the benefits of eating frequently as outlined in the Grazing is good (see pages 26–29). It is easy to adapt this schedule to your daily routine by simply sliding the meal times an hour or so earlier if you are an early riser who has breakfast at 6am, for instance, or slide in the other direction if you commonly eat breakfast at 9am.

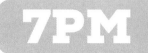

DINNER
rounding off the day

Often there's more time to prepare a meal at the end of the day, so now is your chance to pick and choose your recipe. Leaf through the Main meals section (see pages 140–221) and decide which variation you're going to make tonight.

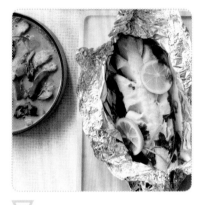

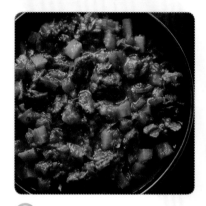

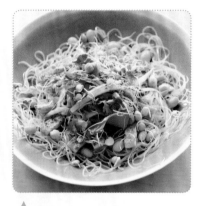

Burn To continue all the great work you've done during the day, try to minimise your carb intake in the evenings. During the evening when you are resting, your body will be predominantly using fat as an energy source. If you add carbs to the mix at this time of the day, they will slowly be converted to body fat as only a small percentage will be used as an energy source. So, opt for Chicken noodle tom yum broth (see page 171) or Thai red fish curry (see page 207).

Balance Unless you have been exercising after work, try to keep away from a carb-heavy meal. A small serving of carbs in this meal isn't the end of the world, but opt for a small handful as opposed to a big serving. Great meals to end your day on this diet code include Hungarian beef goulash and rice (see page 187) and Mackerel masoor dahl (see page 199).

Build If you played sport or exercised after work, then this meal needs to be designed to facilitate recovery and support muscle growth. It also has to see you through the night, so what you need is a high-carb, low-GI meal with a good serving of protein to help promote muscle growth overnight. If you have trained earlier in the day, and not in the evening, the carbohydrate content here will not as important, and may lead to fat storage, so opt for a Balance meal.

Top tip Having a serving of slow-release protein (casein) before sleep can help maintain muscle overnight by drip feeding the muscles with protein. Add half a scoop of casein powder to a 100–150g (scant ½–⅔ cup) serving of low-fat cottage cheese or Greek yogurt with berries or drink in a glass of skimmed milk an hour before bed.

A visual approach to eating

Being aware of calories can have its place in a diet, but adding up all the calories in a recipe or in a snack can become boring and time consuming. Of course, counting calories can be relatively easy if you eat pre-packed foods, as these by law have to have various items of nutritional information on the package (such as energy, carbohydrate, sugar, fat, saturated fat and salt). But there is very little good nutrition in such foods.

The best move you can make when changing to a healthier way of eating is to ditch all processed and pre-packaged foods and instead buy fresh ingredients and cook from scratch. If you're cooking recipes from scratch, working out how many calories a dish or snack contains can start to become a complicated and long-winded process, as fresh ingredients are not labelled with the calorie or macronutrient content (although wouldn't it be great if a carrot, slice of cheese or banana had a magical calorie label on it?). When cooking with fresh ingredients and creating delicious dishes of your own, the only way to quickly calculate calories is to use a dietary analysis software or an app, such as MyFitnessPal.

But you can avoid calorie counting if you follow one of the three diet codes in the book – we've already done the hard work for you, so you can pick and choose whichever dishes you like, with its tailored variation, rather than having to worry about how many grams of flour you're using or how many millilitres of milk. That said, if you can start to monitor how many calories and how much fat or protein an ingredient has, then you'll be on the road to becoming more nutrient savvy and be able to achieve your dietary goals easier and faster.

In this section, we'll show you how visual cues can ensure you're eating the right amount of food and also the right proportions of different foods.

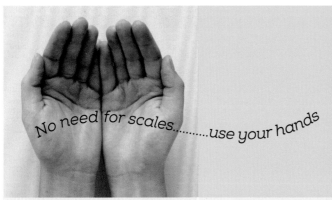

No need for scales..........use your hands

A good way to approach portion control is to use your hands. Generally speaking, the smaller you are the smaller your hands will be; the larger you are the larger your hands. Using hands for portion sizes can be useful as smaller people tend to require fewer calories and nutrients and smaller portions than larger people. A fist equals the amount to match your formed fist; a handful is the amount that fits inside your open hand.

▽ BURN
→ A fist of protein
→ Two handfuls of vegetables or salad (or more if you can fit it on!)
→ A small palm of fat-based foods or 1–2 tsp of oil

◯ BALANCE
→ A fist of protein
→ A handful or two of vegetables or salad
→ A handful of carbohydrate
→ A small palm of fat-based foods or 1–2 tsp of oil

△ BUILD
→ A fist of protein
→ A fist or two of vegetables or salad
→ Two handfuls of carbohydrate
→ One or two palms of fat-based foods or 2–3 tsp of oil

Portion size matters

Research has shown that plate size has increased over 20 per cent since the 1960s; and this equates to people eating much more at each meal than in earlier decades. The super-size nature of the modern world has meant that many people are now super-sized themselves – not a healthy position at all. The size of your plate or bowl has been shown to contribute to the amount of food you eat during a meal. This phenomenon, known as the Delboeuf illusion (see below), was expanded in 1960s to help explain the over-indulging nature of the Western diet. The basis of the illusion is that when a circle (in this case, the circle is food) is placed inside a much larger circle, the inner circle appears smaller than when placed inside a circle only slightly larger.

With the crockery trend leaning towards larger restaurant-style white plates, it can mean that you end up eating more at each meal as the illusion prompts you to think you've not eaten as much as you have. With a smaller plate size, you can easily reduce the amount you eat while your brain sees a full plate being offered. So by switching to smaller plates, the illusion may help you improve portion control and also curb hunger as your brain sees the food as a larger portion than it really is.

Use this illusion to your advantage by opting for a smaller plate when reducing weight (Burn), a normal-sized plate when maintaining weight (Balance) and a larger plate when increasing muscle mass or gaining weight (Build).

Plate sizes

Choose your plate size to match to your diet code to help you give yourself visually the right amount of food for a meal and to fool your brain in to thinking you're eating more than you actually are.

Burn ~21cm (8¼in)

Balance ~24cm (9½in)

Build ~27cm (10¾in)

The inner circle on the right appears bigger but is the same as on the left; this is the Delboeuf illusion.

All proteins are equal, well mostly

Chicken – 25% protein

Beef – 25%

Lamb – 25%

Turkey – 24%

Salmon – 20%

Pulses – 19–24%

White fish – 18–21%

Cheese – 14–28%

Nuts – 14–21%

Grains – 14–18%

Eggs – 13%

Edamame – 11%

Cottage cheese and yogurt – 10–12%

Tofu - 8%

When we talk about protein, we mean meat, poultry, fish and seafood, beans and peas, eggs, soya produce, dairy produce, nuts and seeds (see also page 14). All dishes – whichever diet code you follow – should have a fist-sized portion of protein, which will provide you with roughly the right serving per meal.

All lean-meat-based proteins, such as chicken and beef, contain roughly a similar percentage of protein (see illustration left) and calorie content, so a standard portion size of a fist can be used for all proteins. Oily fish, such as mackerel and salmon, often have slightly lower protein contents and higher calories, but go for the same fist serving size and only include these in your diet three to four times per week (pregnant and breastfeeding women or those trying to get pregnant should limit their intake to twice a week). Other protein sources, such as dairy products and soya products offer varying levels of protein (see left). That said, a fistful of protein should be enough of all these proteins and the recipes are designed to provide your body with just what you need.

Fats – grab a spoon to help

As you might recall, fats come in unsaturated or saturated forms (see also page 18). Unsaturated fats are found in sunflower, rapeseed (canola), olive and vegetable oils, avocados, nuts and seeds and oily fish, whereas you'll find saturated fats in fatty meat and meat products, dairy produce, pastries, cakes, biscuits (cookies), chocolate, coconut oil and palm oil. You've seen earlier and above how easy it is to estimate the protein content of a meal and carbs are simple too (see opposite). Working out the fat content of a meal can be a little bit more difficult as fats can be hidden within other ingredients. Using your hands to measure fats may be a little bit more difficult

(unless you like oil all over your kitchen surfaces and not in your meal!), so grab yourself a more conventional measuring utensil instead – a teaspoon is perfect. You should have a serving of fat with each meal. If you are cooking an oily fish or a fattier cut of meat you won't need an extra serving of fat as there will be enough fat within the fish or meat. But if you are using a leaner cut of meat or a lean-type of meat, such as turkey or chicken, or making a vegetable-based dish, try to incorporate some oil into your dish as a dressing or for cooking (ideally extra virgin olive oil or coconut oil) or top off with a portion of nuts and seeds, for example, or serve with half an avocado on the side.

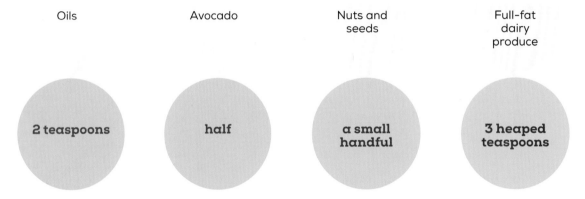

Oils	Avocado	Nuts and seeds	Full-fat dairy produce
2 teaspoons	half	a small handful	3 heaped teaspoons

A spectrum of carbohydrates

Carbohydrates, as you might recall (see also page 16), can be simple (such as sugars, including fruit and milk) and complex (for example starches, including bananas, barley, beans, breads, cereals, chickpeas, flour, lentils, nuts, oats, pasta, potatoes, root vegetables, sweetcorn and yams). Carbohydrate content varies quite a lot between different carbohydrate sources. For example, grains or those foods made from grains (such as rice, quinoa, pasta and couscous) tend to have the highest carbohydrate content – 70–80 per cent, dropping to a much lower amount in root vegetables, for example, where it's 10–20 per cent – see the spectrum of carbs on the right. Due to this, trying to recognise which to add more of and which to cut down on will be essential to controlling both carbohydrate and calorie intake.

Rice noodles - 83% carbs
Rice - 80%
Couscous - 77%
Pasta - 75%
Oats - 66%
Quinoa - 64%
Chickpeas - 61%
Pinto beans - 61%
Kidney beans - 60%
Lentils - 60%
Sweet potato - 20%
Potato - 18%
Butternut squash - 12%
Carrot - 10%

Visual portion sizes for carbs

The chart below shows guidelines for portioning that you should be aiming for when sticking to Burn, Balance or Build meals. Instead of having to weigh everything out, these 'handy' portion sizes will be a quick and easy way of working how many carbs you need.

Breakfasts (mostly in handfuls)

	▽	○	△
Oats	0–½	1	2
Muesli	0–½	1	2
Granola	0–½	1	2
Baked beans	0	½ cup	1 cup
Bread	0	1 slice	2 slices
Potatoes	0	1 potato	2 potatoes

Lunches and dinners (all in handfuls)

	▽	○	△
Rice (dry)	0–½	1	2
Quinoa (dry)	0–½	1	2
Couscous (dry)	0–½	1	2
Pasta (dry)	0–½	1	2
Lentils (dry)	0–½	1	2
Chickpeas (dry)	0–½	1	2
Pulses (dry)	0–½	1	2
Potatoes	1	2	3
Sweet potato	1	2	3
Root vegetables	1	2	3

Clean and natural foods

There are a few simple changes you can make to the foods you choose to buy that will bring about a great difference to your health and vitality. If we had to sum it up in one sentence it would be:

Choose food that's been grown with care, as locally to your home as possible, organically if possible, and cook from scratch, rather than buy highly processed convenience foods.

Quality comes first

Whichever of the diet codes you choose to follow – Burn, Balance or Build or, in fact, if you decide to mix and match – the first step to making any of our mouth-watering recipes is to pay attention to the quality of the foods that you buy and eat.

Many people do much of their food shopping at supermarkets, which have expanded their offer of convenience foods that can be cooked quickly in the microwave for a 5-minute supper in a plastic tray – with all the added preservatives, processed fats and limited nutrition that go with that.

Quality is not always the supermarkets' priority as they seek quantity at the best price, and so quality can suffer with lower-quality produce filling their shelves at low-cost prices. However, many supermarkets do have an organic section where you can find fruits and vegetables that haven't been sprayed with harmful chemicals and preservatives and meats that aren't mass produced and loaded with unnecessary extras.

So, change your approach to food shopping to gain great health benefits. Seek out local specialist shops – the butchers, fishmongers, bakers and greengrocers are returning to our towns and villages or reappearing at weekly farmer's markets – where the provenance of your food can be explained and the quality can be assured.

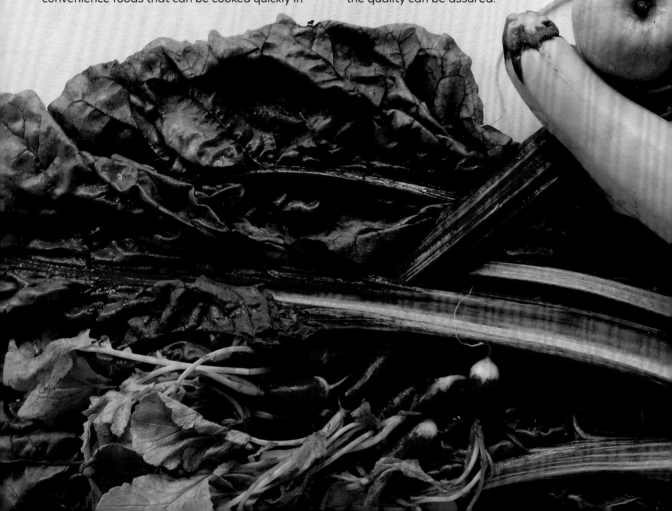

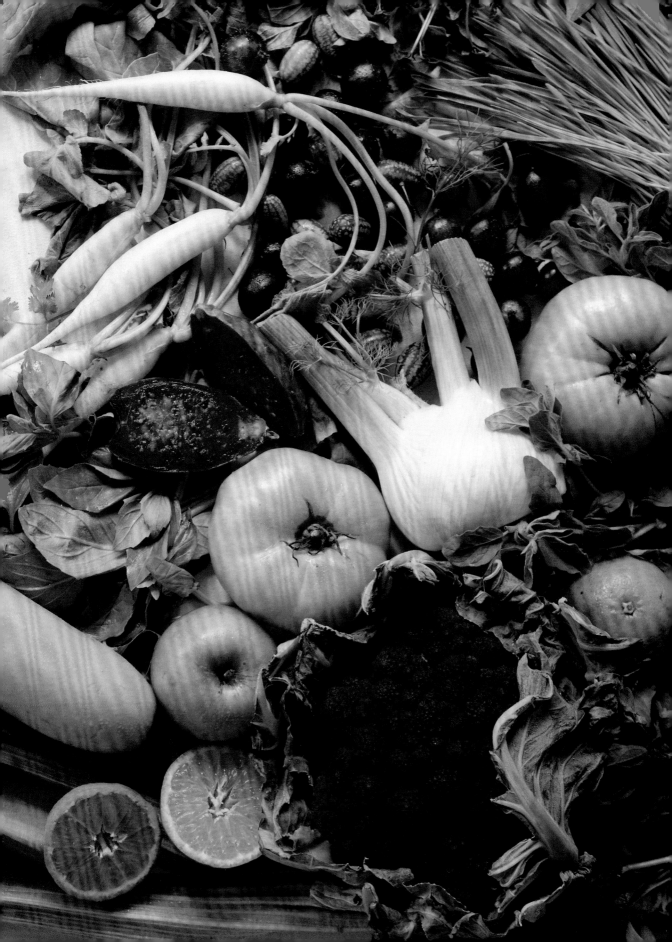

Sourcing your food carefully

Have you ever compared the taste of a supermarket tomato with a home-grown or locally sourced alternative? Give it a go and we can guarantee that you'll agree the difference is staggering. But it is not only the taste that is better, but also the nutrient density of the food.

You can't get more local than your own garden or windowsill. Growing your own produce can't be beaten in terms of both taste and nutrition; it is easy to grow lettuces and herbs in window boxes, tomatoes and mange tout (snow peas) in grow bags and fill gaps in your garden's borders with onions, broad (fava) beans or whatever else you fancy. So, be inspired and just grow one thing to start with; once you've got the bug, you'll buy more seed packets than you'll know what to do with!

The cost of cheap meat and fish

A common misconception of non-organic meats is that hormones are used during production. In fact, in the 1980s, the European Union introduced a ban on using hormones in animals and on imports with traces of hormone residue, meaning all meats farmed or eaten in the EU will be hormone-free.

This is obviously good news, but mass-produced meat goes through a series of processes before it reaches the supermarket shelves. Much of the meat is plumped up with water to make the cut of meat look bigger and weigh more – thereby costing you more. How many times have you cooked an inexpensive chicken breast only to find it noticeably shrink in size during cooking and in the process fill the pan with water? Compare this with a top-quality chicken breast and the difference is clear. In reality, the cheaper chicken breast may actually end up costing more by the time you've finished cooking it, if you measure it gram for gram. And tastewise, it just won't compare.

Farmed fish are subject to far worse conditions than land-reared animals. They are packed in together with many more fish than those ever found in the wild; for instance, each salmon is given the equivalent space of a bath tub of water in a cage with 50,000 other fish. Such intense and inhospitable breeding conditions mean that skin, fin and tail damage is common, as well as disease, parasites and stress. To combat this many antibiotics, hormones and nerve toxins are used. At Soulmatefood, we choose open-water fish, caught on a line and organic where possible.

Become a more savvy shopper. If you choose your foods wisely, the foods you buy will:

→ promote vitality and health

→ contain a wide range of different nutrients

→ have natural enzymes that work for your digestion, not against it

→ be free of trans fats and other hydrogenated fats that can be detrimental to your body.

We think an easy way to cover all of these bases is to:

→ buy organic fruits and vegetables or at least wash all produce before cooking and eating (when in doubt choose foods that have a natural skin, such as bananas, potatoes and kiwis; the skin can act as a natural 'wrapper' keeping out the chemicals used and preserving the inner food)

→ buy all meat and fish locally – this will ensure a better-quality product and choose line-caught/non-farmed fish and grass-fed meat whenever possible as they are more nutritious

→ avoid buying any foods that have a long shelf life; with a few exceptions, these foods tend to be heavily processed and packed full of oils, sugars and preservatives.

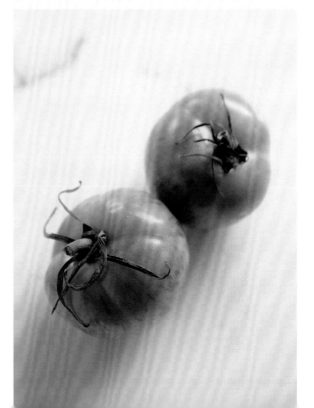

Eating plans
for specific goals

If you have one of the specific goals outlined on the right then you can follow the example diet codes in this section that give you guidelines on which versions of meals and snacks to eat and when. If, for instance, you want to lose some weight or refine your body shape then choose the Eat to manage weight diet code. If you're training for a marathon, obstacle challenge or triathlon, then Eat to toughen up is the code for you. Generally, as you'll soon see, the diet code you follow on days when you're exercising or training is different from the other days – so you're fuelled for your activity.

Eating plans:

Eat to manage weight – p.44

Eat to keep healthy – p.47

Eat to build your body – p.50

Eat to toughen up – p.53

Eat to play team sports – p.57

How hard are you working?
This chart can help you work out what intensity you're working at.

LEVEL OF INTENSITY	HEART RATE (BEATS PER MINUTE)	HOW IT FEELS	WHAT YOUR BODY'S DOING
Low	68–92	Easy	No real sweating unless it's hot and humid. Your breathing remains the same.
Moderate	93–118	Somewhat hard	After about 10 minutes, you'll break a sweat. Your breathing becomes deeper and more frequent. Chatting is possible.
High	›119	Hard	You'll break into a sweat within 5 minutes. Your breathing becomes deep and rapid and it's hard to talk except in brief bursts.

Eat to **manage weight**

It's easy to gain weight through overindulgence or falling off the exercise wagon, but it's great to know that the Burn diet code recipes can help you lose weight and gain vitality while eating totally delicious and easy-to-make dishes. If you're already an active person and want to refine your body shape, then all the Burn versions of the recipes are going to help you achieve your goals, too.

Ditch the fat, keep the muscle

Obviously by following a weight-management plan the ultimate goal will be weight loss, but should weight loss be the only consideration? We think the most important factor should really be *fat loss* not weight loss (which would include both body fat and muscle mass loss). So, the aim of our Eat to manage weight plan is to maximise body fat loss while, at the same time, maintaining muscle mass. As we mentioned earlier (see page 27), muscle tissue is a highly metabolically active tissue. Therefore, by focusing on keeping your muscle mass constant you will further help body fat loss by lessening the reduction in metabolic rate associated with weight loss.

At Soulmatefood, when we think of managing weight a few instances spring to mind:

those looking to lose body fat to improve their health

those in search of the perfect beach body

those involved in weight-categorised combat sports

athletes or sportspeople needing to reduce body fat for body composition goals.

Go for the burn

So, to maximise your body fat loss you'll mostly want to choose the Burn option of each recipe and you can eat mouthwatering foods safe in the knowledge that they're designed with your goal in mind – slimming down. The high protein content of these meals will help to maintain that all-important lean muscle mass by feeding your muscles with amino acids and will also curb your hunger. The only time to switch to a Balance version of a dish is when you're taking part in activity or exercise – in such cases, eat a Balance dish 3–4 hours before your exercise session to fuel your activity.

Setting goals

The most important factor for successful weight loss is to set yourself achievable goals in the short, medium and long term. By setting unachievable and unrealistic goals, you are only setting yourself up to fail from the outset. This is our goal timeline:

> ***short-term goal*** (week to week goals)
> aim to lose 1–2lb (0.5–1kg) per week
> ***medium-term goal*** (within three months)
> aim to lose 1 stone/14lb (6.5kg)
> ***long-term goal*** (within a year)
> aim to lose 2–3 stone/26–42lb (12–19kg).

There has been a lot of research that has shown that the slower the rate of weight loss, the greater the amount of lean muscle maintained – and this is the best way to slim down. The Burn variations when combined together will help you undereat the recommended calorie intake by about 500 kcal per day. Don't worry you won't need to count calories – we've done all that for you; but basically eating the Burn diet code reduces how much you eat by roughly 20–25 per cent. In fact, a simple way of shedding 500 kcal per day would be to avoid

Weight loss *A desk-based worker training three times a week*

	MONDAY	TUESDAY	WEDNESDAY	THURSDAY	FRIDAY	SATURDAY	SUNDAY
Training							
BREAKFAST	▽	▽	▽	▽	▽	▽	▽
Training							
MORNING SNACK	▽	▽	▽	▽	▽	▽	▽
Training							
LUNCH	○	▽	▽	▽	○	▽	▽
Training							
AFTERNOON SNACK	○	▽	▽	▽	○	▽	▽
Training	▬		▬		▬		
DINNER	▽	▽	▽	▽	▽	▽	▽

Slim down *Weight management for a boxer, training five days a week*

	MONDAY	TUESDAY	WEDNESDAY	THURSDAY	FRIDAY	SATURDAY	SUNDAY
Training	▬	▬	▬	▬	▬		
BREAKFAST	▽	▽	▽	▽	▽	▽	▽
Training							
MORNING SNACK	▽	▽	▽	▽	▽	▽	▽
Training							
LUNCH	○	○	▽	○	○	▽	▽
Training							
AFTERNOON SNACK	○	○	▽	○	○	▽	▽
Training	▬	▬		▬	▬		
DINNER	▽	▽	▽	▽	▽	▽	▽

EXERCISE INTENSITY	LOW	MEDIUM	HIGH
	▬	▬	▬

heavily processed fats and refined carbohydrates, something you'll be doing anyway with the Soulmatefood recipes.

Stick with the plan

Don't expect change overnight. You have to show commitment to a plan over a sustained period of time. In contrast, you may step on the scales after a week of the latest fad or crash diet and notice a high rate of weight loss. But what the scales won't be telling you is that this weight loss will predominantly be fluid and muscle, with minimal body fat lost at all. What's more, crash diets over time can reduce your resting metabolic rate due to their effect on reducing muscle mass, which will work against you trying to lose more weight. Increase the chances of staying on the weight-loss wagon by aiming to drop 1–2lb (0.5–1kg) per week.

Track your progress

It's a good idea to have a tangible record to plot your progress over the coming months, so keep a log of your weight on a weekly basis – weigh yourself once a week at the same time on the same day – and when you look back over the months you'll be able to see how well you are doing! There are apps for this kind of log taking but a simple pen and paper record works just as well.

Another good tactic is to take photos every week; why not make Monday photo day? Try to wear the same kinds of clothes each time for the photo, so you can see the changes at a glance. Be aware that if you have started a new exercise regime, when previously you were sedentary, it is possible that initially you may gain weight due to increasing the mass of your newly flexed muscles. Gradual changes easily go unnoticed in the mirror, so by comparing photos week to week and later month to month you will be able to see huge improvements in your body. Such improvements will further boost your mood and confidence.

Keep it real

Have a cheat meal. Yes, you read that right. A cheat meal – that is a non-Burn version of a meal (Balance or Build, whichever you prefer) – once a week is going to do very little harm in the long run and serves as a great reward for all your healthy eating habits the rest of the week.

Specialist slimming for sports

Although fat loss is preferable to weight loss, some people, for instance boxers needing to make a certain weight by a certain time, may even need to reduce muscle mass as well as body fat. If this applies to you, you should reduce your protein intake by roughly a third and replace this with fats or carbs – you'll still need to consume the same number of calories, just fewer of them as protein (25 per cent less). As neither fat nor carbs have an effect on the rate of protein synthesis, this means you will start to lose muscle mass, if required.

HERE ARE SOME BASIC POINTERS

→ Choose the Burn variations of recipes.

→ Reduce your general sugar intake.

→ Reduce your carbohydrate intake and opt for low-GI alternatives where possible.

→ Increase your protein intake – it'll help you feel fuller for longer and use up more calories simply digesting your food.

→ Fill up on vegetables and salad.

→ Try to have healthy snacks to hand when you're out and about to stop you snacking on convenience food when hunger pangs occur.

→ Keep hydrated – try to drink at least 2 litres (8 cups) of water per day (throughout the day) and have a bottle with you at all times. Thirst is easily confused with hunger, so don't automatically reach for food as you could simply be thirsty.

→ Don't be scared of fats. Fats are vital for many metabolic functions. Ingredients such as nuts, seeds, extra virgin olive oil and oily fish are all great examples of fats to include in your diet, just eat them in moderation.

Eat to **keep healthy**

If you're a moderately active person who wants to improve their health and vitality further and aims to do this through the foods you eat, then read on. Below we'll show you which foods are key to achieving this goal and show how following the diet code makes eating nutritious and delicious meals your new route to feeling great.

Not everybody who wants to try a new way of eating wants to lose weight or gain weight; in our experience at Soulmatefood, a great many people want to maintain their weight yet eat in a more healthy way. In our society, many people eat healthily when on a weight-loss diet but as soon as they reach their target weight and are hoping to maintain their new weight, they often, unintentionally, eat less healthily (now the diet is over and they go back to old, less healthy eating habits), which ultimately leads to weight gain. Why switch to eating and drinking junk foods after a healthy 'weight loss' regime? You'll only end up putting the weight back on again. By following the recipes in this book, you can eat tasty and nutrient-packed meals all the time, helping you to maintain weight without falling into the 'diet trap'. A few well-deserved treats here and there are perfectly fine, this isn't the diet police, but paying a little bit more attention to the foods you eat could save you the challenge and hassle of trying to lose weight once again in the future.

Eat carbs for a reason
As you'll see in many of the eating plans in this book, when you eat carbs is vital to maintaining body weight. As a rule of thumb, eat carbs when you are going to be doing exercise and avoid them when you won't be. That doesn't mean cutting them out completely when you are not working out, just limit your intake to a small fist-sized portion in your meals as opposed to a large heap (see A visual approach to eating, page 36).

And when you're eating carbs, choose the high-GI versions (such as Orange and ginger flapjacks, see page 120 or the Coco choc crunch cereal, see page 66) around your activities and the lower-GI options at other times (such as quinoa,

potatoes, sweet potatoes, brown rice, lentils, beans and wholemeal (wholewheat) pasta; see page 16); think of Parmigiana di melanzane (see page 176) or Saffron-poached chicken, barberry rice and baba ganoush (see page 162). When planning what to eat, try to include nutrient-dense ingredients – pack your plates full of colourful vegetables on a daily basis, and stick to eating fruits, such as bananas, strawberries or raisins, to fuel exercise.

Boost your immunity
Foods can have a large impact on your immunity and overall health. If you've often suffered in the past from feeling under the weather or are always likely to catch the latest cold or bug, then once you're following a diet code, you'll find that your health and immunity improve – no more sick days for you!

INVEST IN A GOOD WATER BOTTLE

Drinking enough water through the day is the best way to keep your body hydrated (see also pages 22–25). Sip water constantly during the day; just downing a 500ml (18oz) drink with meals is not the best strategy. Remind yourself to drink regularly by having a water bottle handy at all times. At Soulmatefood, we use clear 500ml (18oz) water bottles and drink at least four of these during the day, and a whole bottle extra for every hour of exercise. Choose clear bottles rather than solid or coloured ones, so that you can see at a glance how much you have drunk.

An active person taking a mixture of exercises, such as yoga and zumba

	MONDAY	TUESDAY	WEDNESDAY	THURSDAY	FRIDAY	SATURDAY	SUNDAY
Training							
BREAKFAST	○	○	○	▽	△	○	▽
Training	▬				▬		
MORNING SNACK	○	○	○	▽	△	○	▽
Training							
LUNCH	○	○	○	▽	○	○	▽
Training				▬			
AFTERNOON SNACK	○	○	△	▽	▽	▽	▽
Training		▬	▬				
DINNER	○	○	△	▽	▽	▽	▽

An active person doing weight training and running

	MONDAY	TUESDAY	WEDNESDAY	THURSDAY	FRIDAY	SATURDAY	SUNDAY
Training							
BREAKFAST	○	○	△	○	○	○	▽
Training			▬				
MORNING SNACK	○	○	△	○	○	○	▽
Training							
LUNCH	○	○	○	▽	○	○	▽
Training							
AFTERNOON SNACK	△	△	○	▽	△	△	▽
Training	▬	▬			▬	▬	
DINNER	△	△	○	▽	△	△	▽

EXERCISE INTENSITY	LOW	MEDIUM	HIGH
	▬	▬	▬

SCALES ARE YOUR FRIEND

Don't be afraid of the bathroom scales, they can help you stay on track. While you don't want to measure your weight on a daily basis, weighing yourself once a week (be sure you do it at the same time of day, ideally in the morning after going to the toilet and before eating or drinking anything) will help you to understand how your body weight normally fluctuates and will help you spot a trend in an upward or downward direction. The theory is simple: if you weigh more than last week, reduce your food intake slightly; if you weigh less, then increase how much you eat. Using scales regularly can motivate you to make smaller changes more often, instead of a huge one when you haven't stepped on them for several months and realise you are far from where you want to be.

It pays to try to eat more than the 'five-a-day' portions of fruit and vegetables, as recent research suggests that it may not be enough. Eating a full complement of the vitamins and minerals in fresh fruit and vegetables is a great approach, but do make sure you're eating a good range of these (in terms of colours) and do not just stick to your favourite couple of fruits or vegetables. The different vitamins and minerals found in fruit and vegetables are what give them their colours, so eating a lot of orange vegetables (such as orange peppers and butternut squash) may give you a good beta-carotene intake but may mean that you're missing out on the iron, calcium and vitamin K found in green, leafy vegetables. Some foods, such as onions, garlic and honey, have antibacterial properties that can also help to reduce the risk of coughs and colds.

Don't beat yourself up over indiscretions

It's perfectly ok to have a cheat meal every now and then (see page 46) or if you find yourself hungry and needing food when there are no healthy options available. Don't feel bad or beat yourself up if you do this occasionally. Simply compensate for it at your next meal by choosing a lower-calorie option or excluding the carbs.

Maintaining a healthy body weight and eating well is about achieving a balance; it's not about counting the calories of every single thing you put in your mouth. Simply put: if you eat more one day, then eat less the next.

Listen to your body

Our bodies do a good job of telling us what it needs and when it needs it, so it's a good idea to listen to it! When you are hungry, eat; when you are not hungry, don't eat! However, make sure you are well hydrated as dehydration can sometimes disguise itself as hunger, meaning that you eat when what your body actually needed was a drink.

HERE ARE SOME BASIC POINTERS

→ Focus on eating Balance versions of the recipes, choosing mostly Build options around training days and Burn dishes on rest days.

→ Aim to eat more than the regular 'five a day' and choose a rainbow of fruits and vegetables.

→ Eat high-GI carbs to fuel exercise sessions and choose low-GI carbs the rest of the time.

→ Keep hydrated – aim to minimise dehydration and make sure you rehydrate properly after activity.

Eat to **build your body**

If you're aiming to increase body strength or bulk up your muscles, then you need to make protein your friend; read on to find out how eating high-protein foods can help you to build more muscles. Combining this knowledge with timed carb intake, increased fat content and an overall increase in calories will help fuel that muscle growth. Below, we show you how to maximise muscle growth.

The main goal of bodybuilding is obviously to increase your body's muscle mass. In order to be able to build muscle, you need to ensure you're eating enough calories so that your body has a positive energy balance and so is ready for building protein not breaking it down. As you'll see from the eating plan (see opposite), five days out of seven is spent eating the Build variations of the recipes; the other two are given over to Balance and Burn for a day apiece.

This approach provides what is known as a positive nitrogen balance while reducing carb intake to limit body fat storage. Without a positive nitrogen balance, muscle mass will break down; increasing protein and therefore amino acids levels increases the nitrogen content of the blood, thereby boosting protein synthesis.

Eat protein to make muscles
Eating at least five servings of protein throughout the day, evenly spaced with 3 or 4 hours between eating, has been shown to maximise muscle protein synthesis (making more muscle); such a high-protein intake will help maintain a positive nitrogen balance (see above) and, therefore, maximise muscle synthesis.

So, you'd have thought that eating protein more often or just more of it would simply emphasise this effect. But no, it's not as simple as that. It appears that optimal protein synthesis seems to require a glut of protein foods followed by low-protein foods for a time and then another glut of protein. Research has shown that when people eat protein at intervals of 3–4 hours it produces a much bigger effect on how much muscle they can make than if the same amount of protein was fed to them continuously via a drip.

Remind yourself how the body makes muscle, see page 14. The research suggests that the mTOR receptors become accustomed to the constant level of protein, which results in them becoming desensitised. So, research backs up the fact that a large hit of protein every 3–4 hours maximises protein synthesis thereby helping you to pack on the pounds, muscle-wise.

Watch the carbs
As we've seen elsewhere (see also Eat to toughen up, page 53), you can eat more carbs to help increase the levels of glycogen (stored energy) in your muscles, which in turn aids training intensity and allows you to increase the load you lift, providing more stress on the muscle to allow for greater growth and adaptation. However, when you increase the carbs you have to deal with the effect of insulin on your blood sugar levels.

To recap, insulin permits sugar to move out of the bloodstream into the cells of the body and allows it to be stored as glycogen (in muscles and the liver). But if there's too much sugar, insulin switches the storage from glycogen to fat. So, be smart about your carb intake by choosing most carbohydrates from the slow-release, low-GI variety, such as brown rice, sweet potato and oats. That said, it's a good idea to fuel any training session with a high-GI intake, such as Apple crumble porridge (see page 76) or Goat's cheese risotto with smoked salmon and beetroot (see page 208) the hour before training as well as up to 30 minutes after training.

WHICH PROTEINS TO CHOOSE?

When you're trying to bulk up and build muscle mass then it pays to know which sources of protein are going to work the best for you. When nutritionists talk of proteins they often refer to slow-release and fast-release proteins; it's a bit like glycaemic index (or GI) for carbs. Some proteins are digested faster, thereby releasing their constituent amino acids more quickly and freeing them up to become future muscle proteins.

Slow-release proteins
Casein (available as a powder to make it fast-release as it doesn't require much digestion) and meats.

Fast-release proteins
Whey and soya (again, in powdered forms make them fast-release as they don't require much digestion).

But it's not just a simple case of eating fast-release proteins all the time for bigger muscles, as you need to stagger your intake of protein throughout the day with a variety of protein sources. Fast-release proteins are great for aiding recovery around training, but we cannot live on protein powders all day, every day. It's best to eat protein from a variety of different sources to ensure you are getting a range of vitamins and minerals in addition to your protein; for example, omega-3 fatty acids from oily fish and iron and zinc from red meat.

Body builder, training four times a week with a session of high-intensity interval training (HIIT)

	MONDAY	TUESDAY	WEDNESDAY	THURSDAY	FRIDAY	SATURDAY	SUNDAY
Training							
BREAKFAST	△	△	○	△	△	△	▽
Training							
MORNING SNACK	△	△	○	△	△	△	▽
Training						▬	
LUNCH	△	△	○	△	△	△	▽
Training							
AFTERNOON SNACK	△	△	○	△	△	△	▽
Training	▬	▬		▬	▬		
DINNER	△	△	○	△	△	△	▽

EXERCISE INTENSITY	LOW	MEDIUM	HIGH

Pile on muscle only

To fuel muscle growth you will need to consume more calories than you burn (see also page 20). However, this can have a negative side – the possibility of gaining body fat. Most people who gain muscle also put on a few pounds of fat. To avoid this we recommend having a reduced-intake day, once a week, where you should eat Burn meals on a non-training or rest day.

Having this low-carb day can help increase fat burning on one day, making sure your waist is not growing faster than your muscles! This low-carb day will also help you make the most of your carbohydrates when you reintroduce these to your diet in the form of high-carb meals around training.

What's more, this technique will help make sure you have enough fuel for your training sessions but and will help reduce the amount of body fat you store when you are not training. The majority of the carbs you eat will be used during training; when refuelling afterwards, the carbohydrates will be forced into the depleted muscles as opposed to being converted to fat.

DRINKING CALORIES – SHAKES AND SMOOTHIES

If you are trying to gain muscle mass or body weight and are already eating plenty of Build meals and snacks but are still not making headway, then it's time to locate a blender. You can drink your calories – take a look at the shake and smoothie recipes (see pages 222–236) and add a scoop of flavoured or unflavoured whey protein or casein powder, if you need an extra protein punch. As well as having fun in the kitchen and using up fruits and/or vegetables that are looking a little past their best, these shakes and smoothies can really pack in the calories, helping you gain more weight.

HERE ARE SOME BASIC POINTERS

→ Focus on eating the Build versions of the recipes, following Balance versions of meals on one non-training day and Burn options for the other day.

→ Eat Build snacks and Build meals 1 hour before and up to 30 minutes after training.

→ Drink shakes and smoothies to make sure you're getting enough calories.

→ Keep hydrated – aim to minimise dehydration and make sure you rehydrate properly after activity. Carb-containing drinks should be consumed before, during and after only very hard sessions or matches, otherwise, stick to water with electrolytes in light-moderate training sessions.

Eat to **toughen up**

When we talk of toughening up, what we mean is preparing your body for endurance. Whether you're setting yourself a challenge of running your first marathon, have got hooked on triathlons or road cycle racing or have signed yourself up to a hard-core obstacle race or endurance event, you'll find plenty of helpful advice on how to feed your body for this type of fitness.

The right type of fuel

Whichever type of endurance race you're preparing for, the basic nutritional principles remain the same: maximising the amount of glycogen in your muscles (see also page 17) to fuel both training and performance at the event.

At Soulmatefood, we realise that people from all walks of life take part in all types of endurance events – from someone with a desk-based job who trains 1–2 hours in the evening and weekends (so about three or four times a week) to elite athletes who train 6+ hours per day – so specific recommendations will vary (see page 55). As a rule of thumb, though, if you are preparing or participating in such events you should be following the Build versions of the recipes most of the time and opting for the Balance versions at times when you're not training. To use the above examples if you're an athlete training 6+ hours a day you should be eating Build meals for every meal, whereas the desk-based worker should choose Balance meals when not training and opt for Build meals 4 hours before training, a Build snack 1 hour before training and a Build meal as soon as possible after training.

Them bones, them bones

Another very important factor to consider in endurance activities is bone health. To keep bones strong and with a healthy bone mineral density (see also page 21), you need to be able to support your own weight during exercise. So, to explain the potential risks you need to be aware of, we have split the types of endurance sport into two categories: high-load and non-weight-bearing.

High-load sports, such as long-distance running, put excessive strain on bones due to the high-impact and repetitive nature of the foot strikes. Over time if you don't take action to protect your bones (see page 54) then you can end up with stress fractures within the bone.

Non-weight-bearing sports, such as cycling or swimming, provide a different problem for bone health as they don't promote bone density and so you can end up with reduced bone density, known as osteopenia (see page 21). Osteopenia is classed as low bone mineral density and is just a step away from osteoporosis. In one research study two-thirds of professional cyclists were osteopenic.

To offset the detrimental effects of non-weight-bearing sports on bone health, try to include weight-bearing exercise, such as running or resistance training, into your exercise schedule at least once per week.

Building strong and healthy bones

So, how can you protect your bones and ensure optimum bone density? The two main micronutrients important for bone health are calcium and vitamin D, so the first step to good

OUR TOP 5 NON-DAIRY SOURCES OF CALCIUM

Kale – 205mg per 100g

Spinach - 153mg per 100g

Chickpeas – 105mg per 100g

Sesame seeds – 95mg per 100g

Chia seeds – 69mg per 100g

CARB LOADING AHEAD OF AN EVENT

In the week before your event, reduce your carbohydrate intake five days away from competition but keep your training levels roughly the same. Over the next few days gradually reduce your carb intake further until on the third low-carb day you avoid carbs altogether. This coupling of training with a reduced carb intake will deplete your muscles and liver of their glycogen stores of energy. Running down your stores of energy like this might seem odd ahead of an event but this depletion promotes a boost of glycogen storage over the remaining two days before the race. So, for the next two days (that is, the two days before the event) you can literally eat as many carbohydrates as you can (see examples on page 56). Cramming in carbs in this way promotes glycogen storage in the muscles and liver. Since you've depleted your muscles of their glycogen stores over the previous three days, they will be much more receptive to an influx of carbohydrates, and as a result they overcompensate and store much more glycogen than would have been stored if there had been no depletion first.

bone health is to eat a diet with plenty of foods rich in these elements. The obvious first stop for calcium-rich foods is dairy produce, such as milk, cheese and yogurts, but don't overlook other non-dairy sources of calcium (see box on page 53). Recipes with bone-building ingredients include 'After Eight' yoatie (see page 72), Granola, berries and vanilla yogurt (see page 62) and Kale dip with sugar snap peas (see page 106).

Vitamin D is also vital for healthy bones as it helps with the absorption of calcium. As 90 per cent of the vitamin D in our body is generated from sunlight, most people should have adequate levels of vitamin D in the summer months, but during winter when the sun's rays are weaker and we expose our skin to the sun less, it might be worth taking a vitamin D supplement; check with your doctor before buying one yourself. You can find vitamin D in certain foods, such as eggs and oily fish, but not enough to provide sufficient vitamin D levels for healthy bones.

Refining your regime for hydration and fuel

During training it is hard to completely stop dehydration, as it's unlikely you will be able to drink at the rate of sweat loss; during competitions there may be more opportunities to drink (such as en-route fluid stations). Remind yourself of the recommendations for hydration (see pages 22–25) to minimise dehydration and maximise rehydration afterwards.

When it comes to fuelling your body for training and an endurance event, you will need to eat enough carbs to maintain energy stores and reduce the chance of 'hitting the wall'. We can store enough glycogen in our muscles (highly trained individuals can store more) to provide fuel for roughly 2 hours' worth of exercise. After this energy store has been depleted, your body turns to fat as a fuel source – and this doesn't feel great when you're taking part in an event: some say that their legs feel like they're going to buckle, their brain's telling them to stop and their body feels heavy. So, use a carb-based sports drink to replace any glycogen and

An obstacle endurance competitor doing two sessions of strength training and two sessions of endurance training a week as well as a weekend event

	MONDAY	TUESDAY	WEDNESDAY	THURSDAY	FRIDAY	SATURDAY	SUNDAY
Training							
BREAKFAST	○	○	▽	○	○	○	▽
Training							
MORNING SNACK	○	○	▽	○	○	△	▽
Training						▬	
LUNCH	△	△	▽	△	△	○	▽
Training							
AFTERNOON SNACK	△	△	▽	△	△	○	▽
Training	▬	▬		▬	▬		
DINNER	△	△	▽	△	△	○	▽

An elite runner training twice a day most days and with one rest day

	MONDAY	TUESDAY	WEDNESDAY	THURSDAY	FRIDAY	SATURDAY	SUNDAY
Training							
BREAKFAST	△	△	▽	△	△	○	▽
Training	▬	▬		▬	▬	▬	▬
MORNING SNACK	△	△	▽	△	△	○	▽
Training							
LUNCH	△	△	▽	△	△	○	▽
Training							
AFTERNOON SNACK	△	△	▽	△	△	○	▽
Training	▬	▬		▬	▬		
DINNER	△	△	▽	△	△	○	▽

EXERCISE INTENSITY	LOW	MEDIUM	HIGH
	▬	▬	▬

supply of fast-release energy gels for energy boosts during an event.

You wouldn't wear brand-new trainers to run a marathon, would you? The same goes for switching what you drink or eat in training or on the day of an event: never try new strategies on the day of a race, get used to them first in training and then once you know they're working you can use them during competitions.

Trying out new high-carb strategies (not to be confused with carb loading, see page 54) in competition may lead to stomach upset and even sickness if you cannot tolerate the carb intake – this is what's known as gastrointestinal or GI distress, see page 21) .

Recovery afterwards

After training or competing in an endurance event, it is vitally important to replace the carbohydrate used as the energy stores will have been severely depleted. Try to eat a high-carb Build meal, such as the Build variation of Parmigiana di melanzane (see page 176) within 30 minutes of finishing training as the muscles will be more receptive within this time window and so can store more glycogen. If this is not possible, opt for a Build snack, such as Ultimate power bar (see page 123), afterwards and then have a Build variation of a meal as soon as possible after that. The Build snacks will also contain a good amount of protein to aid muscle recovery.

fluids lost during the race. The easiest way to do this and to 'kill two birds with one stone' is to use a sports drink that contains 30–40g of carbohydrate per 500ml (18oz) bottle. The drink should also contain electrolytes to aid hydration (this is especially important in hot conditions) so look for sodium, magnesium, potassium and calcium on the packaging for signs of electrolytes. Keep a handy

HERE ARE SOME BASIC POINTERS

→ Focus on eating the Build and Balance versions, with Burn options on non-training or rest days; this strategy will help control body fat levels and better utilisation of carbs when consuming the Build or Balance meals.

→ Eat a Build meal 4 hours before, a Build snack 1 hour before and a Build meal (or a snack if a meal isn't available) immediately after training.

→ Be sure to eat plenty of calcium-rich foods every day (see box on page 53)

→ Use a carb-loading strategy (see page 54) to fuel competition performance.

→ Keep hydrated – aim to minimise dehydration and make sure you rehydrate properly after activity. Carb-containing drinks should be consumed before, during and after only hard sessions, otherwise stick to water with electrolytes in light-moderate training sessions. Aim to drink 500ml (18oz/2 cups) of fluid per hour while training, more in hot conditions (see also pages 22–25).

Eat to **play team sports**

Whether you love to play hockey, football (soccer), rugby or basketball, being involved in any team sport means that you have to tread the fine line between being able to fuel all the training and matches and maintaining a good level of body fat. Get to know your carbs and when to eat and not to eat them, as that's key to becoming the best team player, performance-wise.

In most team sports, you'll have a weekly match or game with training sessions inbetween. So that your body is in the best shape to be able to perform until the whistle blows at full time, you need to learn how much carbohydrate to eat and eat it only at certain times of the week. Don't worry, though, we'll tell you all you need to know about how to do this.

Pre-match nutrition
As with many sports, those playing team sports can range from a Sunday league player who plays once a week and trains once a week, through to elite professionals who play once or twice a week, but who train up to 3 hours a day, three or four times per week. So, depending where you sit on this spectrum, you'll have to adapt what you eat to suit your match and training schedule for the level at which you compete. Hydration is also vital, so remind yourself how much you should be drinking and how often, see pages 22–25.

Your carb intake plays a vital role and getting the balance between too much and too little carbohydrate and at the wrong and right times is essential. At the beginning of the week, you need to be careful, so that your carbohydrate intake just covers the expenditure of training (or even slightly below this). When approaching the weekend, you'll need to boost how much carbohydrate you're eating for two days before the match or game; for example if Saturday is match day then fill up on carbs on Friday and on Saturday morning (see page 59).

ON THE DAY BEFORE A MATCH

→ Eat the Build versions of meals and snacks to boost your carb intake – Beef and vegetable tagine with cauliflower 'couscous' (see page 184) or Pesto and crème fraîche chicken (see page 153) are great dishes.
→ Choose dishes with low-GI, slow-release forms of carbs, such as brown rice, quinoa, couscous, sweet potato, wholemeal (wholewheat) pasta and oats. Try Causa santa rosa (see page 203).
→ Pile fibrous vegetables, such as cauliflower, kale, broccoli and cabbage, on your plate at meals.

GIVE YOURSELF THE EDGE

Chemicals in beetroot, known as dietary nitrates, can temporarily widen blood vessels (vasodilation) in your body, helping it to use oxygen more efficiently and thereby boosting your endurance performance. So, partner your breakfast for two days beforehand and on the morning just before a game with a glass of beetroot containing juice (see pages 229 and 233) or a small concentrated shot of beetroot (such as BeetActive) to take advantage of its vasodilatory benefits. If you're not the biggest fan of beetroot, then you can add the shot to one of the smoothie recipes (see pages 222–236) and you'll get the benefits without the earthiness.

Amateur team sports player training once a week, with one gym session per week and a match on Sunday

	MONDAY	TUESDAY	WEDNESDAY	THURSDAY	FRIDAY	SATURDAY	SUNDAY
Training							
BREAKFAST	▽	▽	▽	▽	▽	△	△
Training							
MORNING SNACK	▽	▽	▽	▽	▽	△	△
Training							(low)
LUNCH	▽	▽	○	△	▽	△	△
Training							
AFTERNOON SNACK	▽	▽	○	△	▽	△	△
Training			(medium)	(medium)			
DINNER	▽	▽	○	△	▽	△	○

Professional team sports player training four times a week with a match on Saturday

	MONDAY	TUESDAY	WEDNESDAY	THURSDAY	FRIDAY	SATURDAY	SUNDAY
Training							
BREAKFAST	○	○	△	▽	△	△	▽
Training							
MORNING SNACK	○	○	△	▽	△	△	▽
Training	(high)	(high)	(high)		(low)		
LUNCH	○	○	△	▽	△	△	▽
Training						(medium)	
AFTERNOON SNACK	▽	▽	▽	▽	△	△	▽
Training							
DINNER	▽	▽	▽	▽	△	△	▽

EXERCISE INTENSITY	LOW	MEDIUM	HIGH

Match day nutrition

In our example below of what to eat on match day, we take a typical amateur football (soocer) player, but the strategies apply to all other team sports. These strategies will help you to maximise the stores of energy (glycogen) in your muscles and liver in order to fuel a full 90 minutes of play, all the way to the final whistle. The timing in this plan is based on a 3pm kick-off so adjust your times forward or push back, as necessary, an hour for every hour of fluctuation.

Breakfast Stock up on carbs and opt for a Build version of breakfast, such as one of the yoaties (see pages 71, 72 and 75) or if you've got time have a cooked breakfast, again following the Build variations. And to give you more energy for later, add a smoothie alongside (see pages 222–236) – it's an easy way of adding in carbs.

3 hours before Eat a slow-release, low-GI carb-based Build meal – such as the Build versions of Keralan rasam (see page 160) or Saffron-poached chicken, barberry rice and baba ganoush (see page 162).

45 minutes before Raise your blood sugar levels by choosing a high-carb, high-GI Build snack such as Violet and raspberry muffins (see page 118) or Orange and ginger flapjacks (see page 120).

At half time Use a carb-based sports drink to replace any glycogen and fluids lost during the match. The easiest way to do this is to use a sports drink containing 30–40g of carbohydrate per 500ml (18oz) bottle. The drink should also contain electrolytes to aid hydration (especially important in hot conditions) so look for sodium, magnesium, potassium and calcium on the packaging for signs of electrolytes. Don't eat any food as it may cause GI distress (see page 21) when the match kicks off again; instead, nibble on an easy-to-digest energy gel to boost energy.

After the match You'll need to rehydrate and eat a wholesome meal as soon as possible after the match. It's a good idea to do some of the prep for your meal beforehand – take one of the Build dishes that works well eaten cold in an airtight container, such as Feta, turkey and warm lentil salad (see page 172). Great snacks include Pesto and polenta protein muffins (see page 119) or Gingerbread bites (see page 112). If you find it hard to stomach food so soon after exertion, make yourself a Build smoothie to have instead (see page 226, 229 and 236), with added whey protein to aid your body's recovery.

HERE ARE SOME BASIC POINTERS

→ Focus on eating the Burn versions of the recipes and switch to Balance meals on training days and ramping up to Build variations of dishes before and after matches. (Professional footballers will have much higher expenditures than amateur team sport players and so they need to switch to Balance dishes on rest days as they need higher carbohydrate stores.)

→ Eat a Build meal 3 hours before and 45 minutes before a match or game.

→ Keep hydrated – aim to minimise dehydration and make sure you rehydrate properly after activity. Carb-containing drinks should be consumed before, during and after only very hard sessions or matches, otherwise, stick to water with electrolytes in light-moderate training sessions.

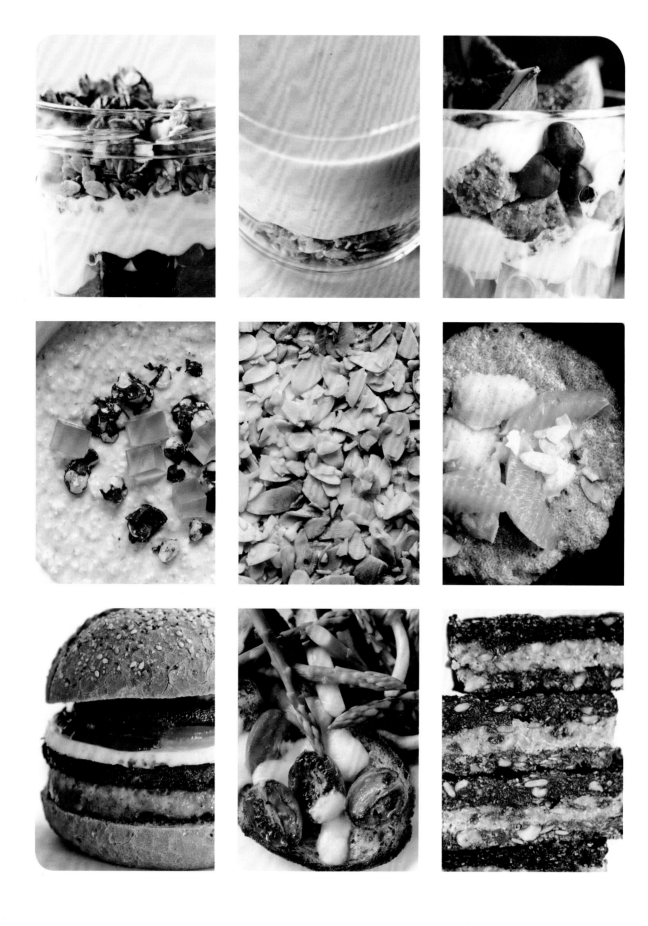

BREAKFASTS

Granola, berries and vanilla yogurt

An oaty breakfast is a great way to start the day. If you're pressed for time in the mornings, then bake a batch of granola and keep in an airtight container (it'll last two weeks or so) – then eat in a matter of minutes.

Health Red and purple berries are a great source of anthocyanins, chemicals that may help to reverse mental decline.

Sport Anthocyanins also can help reduce muscle soreness, thereby aiding recovery after a particularly strenuous training session.

SERVES 4

FOR THE GRANOLA:

150g (1¾ cups) rolled oats

50g (¼ cup) agave syrup

5 tsp sunflower oil

25g (¼ cup) sunflower seeds

25g (¼ cup) pumpkin seeds

25g (1oz) coconut shavings

½ tsp ground cinnamon

FOR THE VANILLA YOGURT:

250g (1 cup) Greek yogurt

50g (2 heaping tbsp) honey

seeds from 1 vanilla pod (bean)

FOR THE BERRIES:

50g (⅓ cup) blackberries

50g (⅓ cup) blueberries

50g (scant ½ cup) raspberries

50g (½ cup) goji berries

Preheat the oven to 180°C/350°F/gas mark 4 and you'll need a baking tray (cookie sheet).

Mix the oats together with the agave syrup and sunflower oil and bake in a baking tray (cookie sheet) in a preheated oven for 10 minutes until golden brown. Stir through the sunflower and pumpkin seeds, coconut shavings and cinnamon and bake for a further 5 minutes.

In a bowl, tip out the yogurt and mix thoroughly with the honey and vanilla seeds so they're well combined.

Divide the berries between 4 bowls, spoon over the yogurt and sprinkle on the granola for texture.

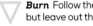 **Burn** Follow the recipe above, but leave out the granola.

 Build Follow the recipe above, and add extra sunflower seeds and dried cranberries (20g/ scant ¼ cup of each per portion) to the granola.

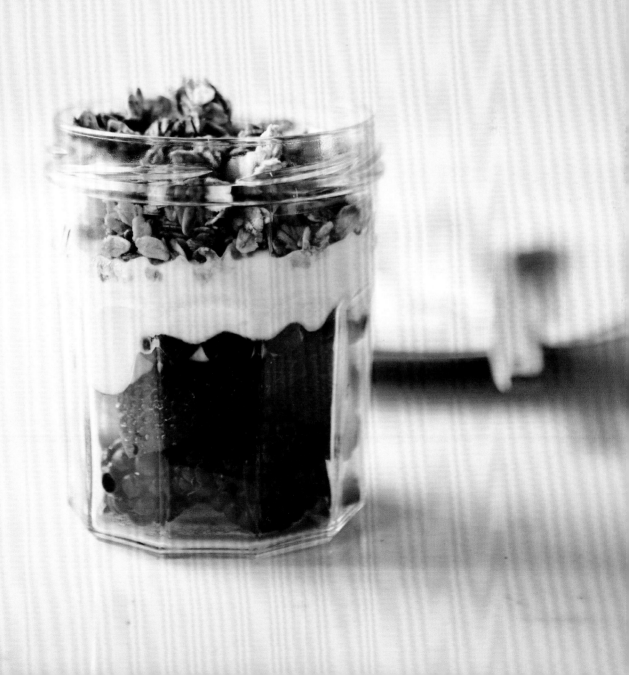

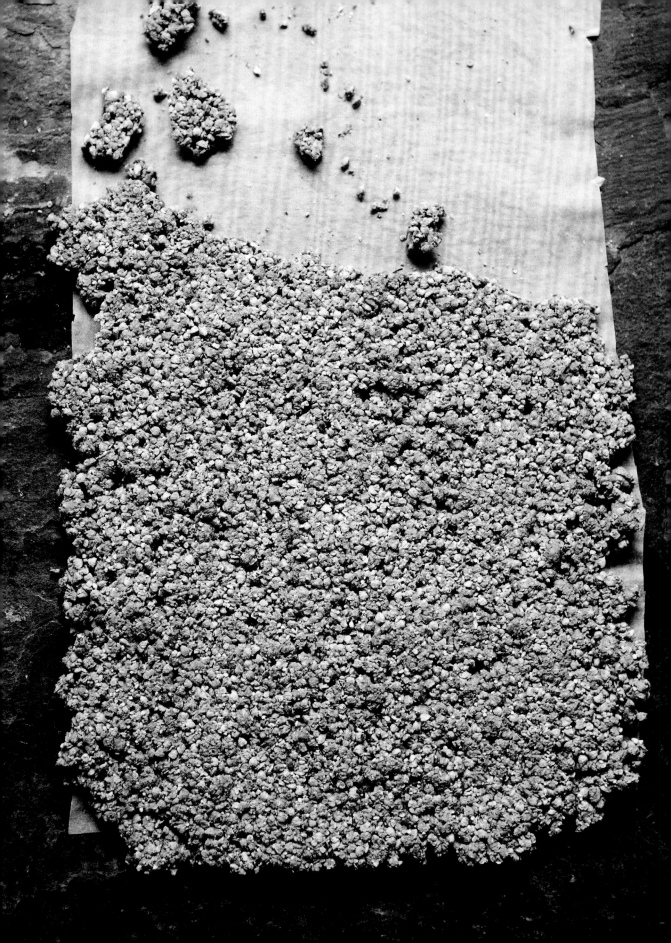

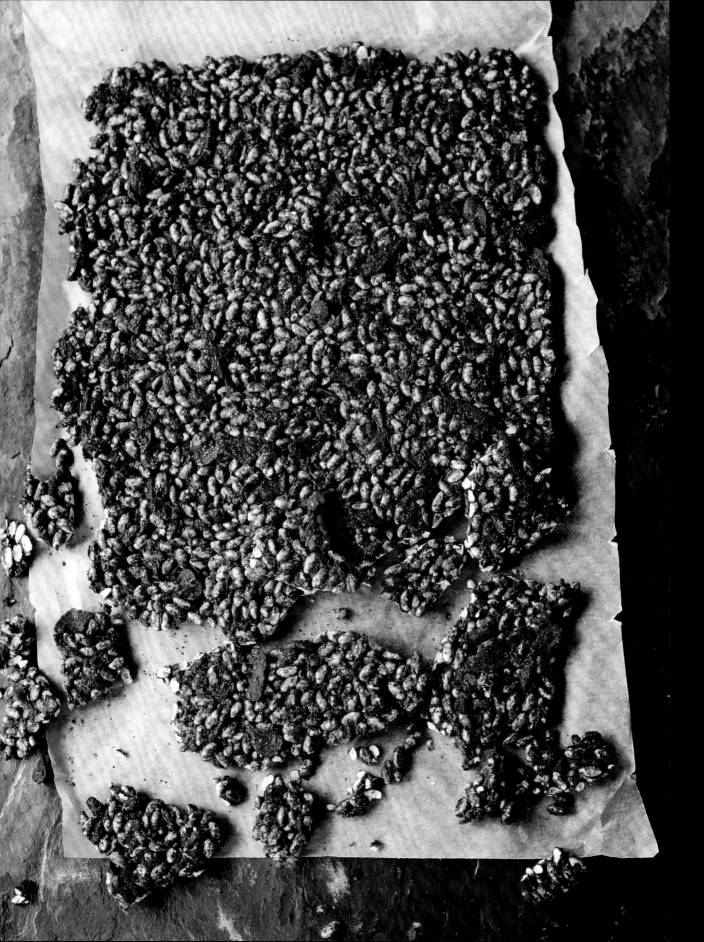

Coco choc crunch

You'll need to keep this cereal on the top shelf or you'll definitely be fighting the kids for it.

Health This cereal is a double winner as it's low in cholesterol and has a low GI.

Top tip This versatile crunch can be enjoyed on top of yogurt, ice cream or on its own as a snack.

FOR THE CEREAL (MAKES 8 PORTIONS):

100g (¼ cup) honey

60g (⅓ cup) coconut palm sugar

12g (2½ tbsp) cocoa powder

30g (⅓ cup) desiccated (dry unsweetened) coconut

100g (½ cup) dried apricots

20g (scant ¼ cup) coconut flour

100g (7 cups) unsweetened puffed rice

FOR THE VANILLA MILK:

25g (1oz) vanilla-flavoured whey protein

120ml (½ cup) semi-skimmed (lowfat) milk

75g (½ cup) blueberries, to serve

▽ **Burn** This dish falls within the 80/20 category (see page 10).

△ **Build** Add 1 sliced banana and 15g (10) hazelnuts per portion.

Preheat the oven to 130°C/266°F/gas mark ½ and you'll need a baking tray (cookie sheet). In a large pan, melt the honey and sugar with the cocoa powder. Bring this to the boil and then simmer for 4 minutes, stirring continuously. Remove the pan from the heat and add the coconut, chopped apricots and flour, using a wooden spoon to mix them thoroughly. While the mixture is still hot, stir in the puffed rice until completely coated.

You'll need 2 sheets of baking parchment. Put 1 on your work surface and spoon out the mixture. Put the second on top and use a rolling pin to spread it out to a thickness of 5–6mm (¼in). Transfer the sandwiched mixture to the baking tray (cookie sheet) and peel off the top sheet. Bake for 50–60 minutes. Pop a saucer in the fridge.

Check the cereal after 50 minutes by pulling off a small piece and putting it on a cold saucer in the fridge for a few minutes. Taste it; it should be crunchy. If it's chewy, pop it back into the oven for a bit longer. When it's done, remove from the oven and allow to cool.

Using a hand-held blender and beaker mix the protein and the milk. Break the sheet into small pieces. To serve a portion, weigh out 40g (1½oz) of the coco choc pieces into a bowl and top with the blueberries and vanilla milk. Store the rest of the cereal in an airtight container, where it will last for 2–3 weeks.

Buckwheat and maple crispies with strawberries

This simple-to-prepare cereal stores for up to two weeks and also makes a fab quick snack. Served here with fresh blueberries and yogurt, it's a truly delicious NY-deli-style breakfast.

Health Buckwheat is a great vegetarian protein source as it has a full amino acid profile, it is also wheat free (despite its name).

Sport The anthocyanins in strawberries can act as potent antioxidants to help combat the oxidative stress caused by exercise.

MAKES 10 PORTIONS

120g (⅓ cup) maple syrup

150g (1 cup) whole buckwheat (aka buckwheat groats)

100g (⅔ cup) pecans, chopped

60g (⅓ cup) quinoa flakes

▽△ **Burn and Build**
Portion size for crispies:
Burn 30g (1oz)
Build 50g (1oz)

Preheat the oven to 120°C/250°F/gas mark ½. Line a baking tray (cookie sheet) with baking parchment. In a small pan bring the maple syrup to the boil then simmer and reduce it by a third. Using a hand-held blender and a beaker, blitz 50g (⅓ cup) of buckwheat to a coarse powder. Put the rest of the buckwheat along with the other dry ingredients into a bowl and pour on the reduced maple syrup.

Tip out the crispie mixture onto the prepared tray and smooth out the surface a little – it should be about 1–1.5cm (½–⅝in) thick. Bake in a preheated oven for 1 hour or until completely dried out. Remove from the oven and allow to cool; break up into bite-sized pieces and store in an airtight container. For a portion, serve 40g (1½oz) crispies in a bowl, with 120g (½ cup) Greek yogurt and 60g (scant ½ cup) fresh strawberries.

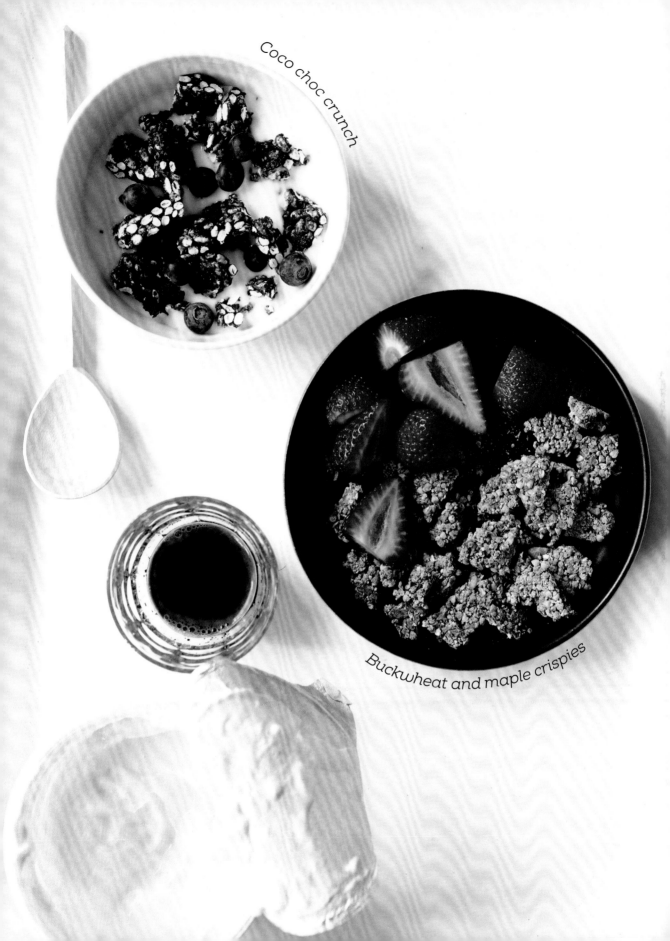

Coco choc crunch

Buckwheat and maple crispies

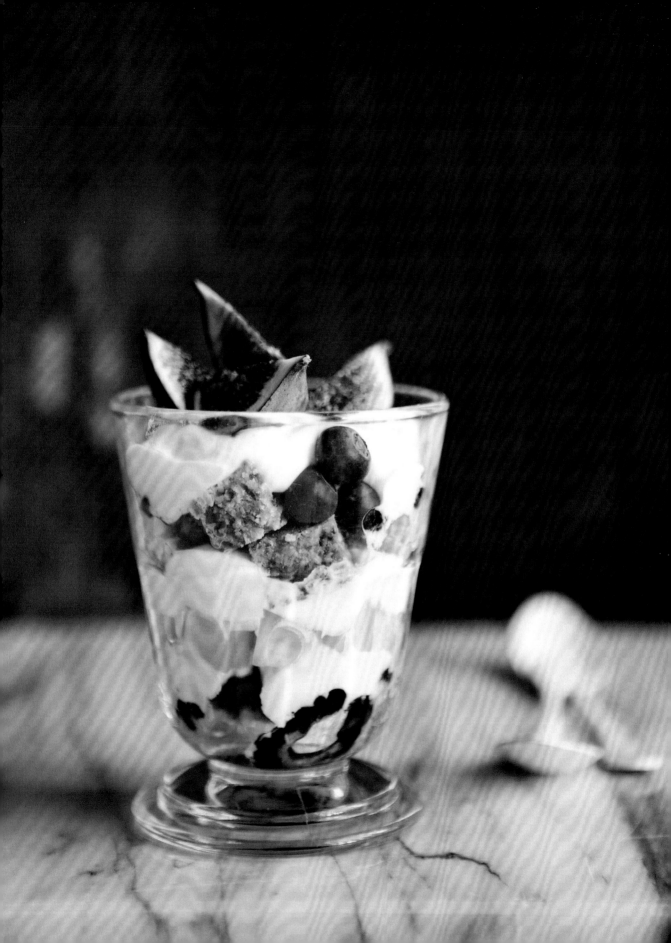

Spiced honey flapjack breakfast sundae

This protein-packed, sweet breakfast is perfect for those with a hectic morning that require refuelling first thing. This sundae can even be made up the night before for an on-the-go nutritional breakfast.

Health The high-fibre oats and figs mean that this breakfast will do wonders for your digestive system.

Sport If you're training in the morning and need a quick carb fix, opt for this breakfast to see you through your activity or to top up the energy banks after a morning workout.

SERVES 2

FOR THE FLAPJACK:

375g (1 cup) honey

375g (1⅔ cups) spreadable light butter

600g (10½ cups) flaked oats

30g (1oz) unflavoured whey protein

¾ tsp ground cinnamon

¾ tsp ground allspice

FOR THE FRUIT:

1 small mango

2 figs

40g (¼ cup) blackberries

40g (¼ cup) blueberries

FOR THE HONEYED YOGURT:

200g (scant 1 cup) Greek yogurt

2 tsp honey

Preheat the oven to 160°C/325°F/gas mark 2½ and line a baking tray (cookie sheet) with baking parchment.

Melt the honey and butter in a large pan on a low heat. Remove from the heat and then add the oats, whey protein and spices, and mix well with a wooden spoon.

Turn the mixture out onto the prepared baking tray (cookie sheet) and bake in a preheated oven for 20–25 minutes until golden brown. Remove from the oven and allow to cool.

When cool, turn the flapjack out onto a chopping (cutting) board and divide into 15 pieces (each should weigh about 80g/3¼oz). One piece makes a portion for a snack. This flapjack keeps for a week in an airtight container.

Next, prepare the fruit. Peel the mango, remove its stone and cut into small cubes. Quarter the figs.

Make the honeyed yogurt by mixing the yogurt and honey together.

To assemble, cut 1 piece of flapjack into small bite-sized cubes. In 2 glasses, create various layers of yogurt, different fruits and flapjack, ending with the fig quarters.

▽ **Burn** Remove the flapjack and replace with 15g (2½ tbsp) pecans per portion.

△ **Build** Increase the flapjack serving to 110g (4oz) and top with 15g (½oz) of your favourite dried fruit.

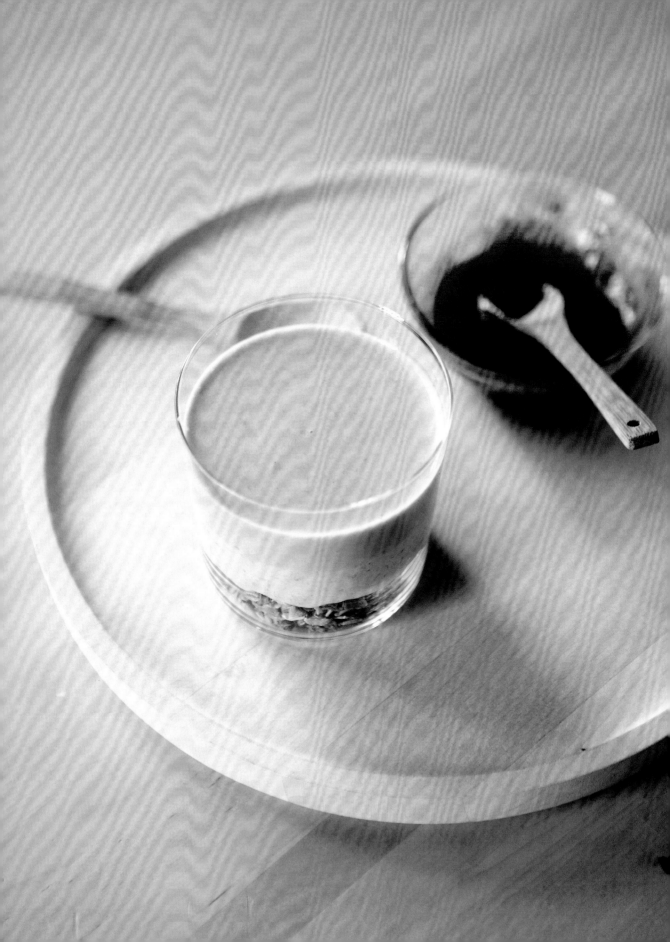

Strawberry cheesecake yoatie

Cheesecake... for breakfast? That's right, we have combined the flavours of the classic dessert with the functionality of a breakfast to give a meal that will go down a treat and fuel your morning's activities.

Sport A favourite of Team GB's boxing squad, who use the breakfast to fuel their morning training sessions or to snack on afterwards to recover.

Top tip Why not make the yoatie base and experiment with different flavour combinations of your own? If you make a good one, share with your friends and also with us!

SERVES 2

FOR THE YOATIE:

90g (1½ cups) flaked oats

140ml (scant ⅔ cup) apple juice

65g (¼ cup) natural yogurt

FOR THE GRANOLA:

85g (⅓ cup) agave syrup

⅓ tsp ground cinnamon

200g (3½ cups) flaked oats

FOR THE COMPÔTE:

170g (generous 1 cup) strawberries

20g (3 tsp) agave syrup

FOR THE CHEESECAKE MIX:

50g (⅓ cup) strawberries

1½ tsp agave syrup

60g (¼ cup) cottage cheese

First, make the yoatie. Mix the oats, apple juice and yogurt together in a bowl, then set aside in the fridge to soak for at least 2 hours (ideally, do this the day before).

Next, make the granola. Preheat the oven to 180°C/350°F/gas mark 4. Mix all the ingredients together until well combined, then tip out onto a non-stick baking tray (cookie sheet) or a tray lined with baking parchment. Bake in a preheated oven for 10–12 minutes until golden. Remove from the oven, allow to cool and set aside. This granola keeps for 2 weeks when stored in an airtight container.

For the compôte, crush the strawberries with the back of a fork and place in a pan with the agave syrup. Bring to the boil over a medium heat, stirring continuously until it starts to thicken – about 2–3 minutes. When done, transfer to a small container and refrigerate.

Lastly, make the cheesecake mix. Place the ingredients into a plastic beaker and blitz until smooth using a hand-held blender. Set aside.

To assemble your yoatie, weigh out 60g (2¼oz) of the granola into the bottom of 2 steep-sided bowls or tumblers (30g/1oz in each). Next, spoon half of the yoatie mix into each bowl, followed by half the cheesecake mix and then top each with the compôte or serve on the side, it's up to you. Enjoy!

Burn Replace the oats, apple juice and yogurt ingredients with 150g (⅔ cup) low-fat Greek yogurt sweetened with 15g (1 tbsp) honey. Use this mixture to replace the yoatie, and layer up with the other ingredients as above.

Balance Reduce the yoatie ingredient quantities to 70g (scant 1 cup) oats, 125ml (½ cup) apple juice and 55g (scant ¼ cup) yogurt.

'After Eight' yoatie

Start the day with something indulgent yet extremely nutritious. Developed for those with a sweeter tooth; this oaty breakfast is our play on a classic flavour combination and delivers just enough of a chocolate hit.

Health This breakfast is brimming with polyphenols (in the dark chocolate), which fight oxidative stress and promote heart health.

Sport This breakfast makes a great low-GI snack. Make a batch and keep refrigerated for a couple of days to use as a post-training recovery snack.

SERVES 2

FOR THE YOATIE:

185g (2¼ cups) rolled oats

280ml (1¼ cups) apple juice

130g (½ cup) natural yogurt

FOR THE NUTTY MIX:

50g (⅓ cup) hazelnuts

30g (1oz) dark chocolate (minimum 70% cocoa solids)

FOR THE JELLY (SERVES 4):

¾ leaf gelatine

40ml (1½ tbsp) apple juice

30g (4½ tsp) agave syrup

peppermint extract

Burn Replace the yoatie part with 150g (⅔ cup) low-fat Greek yogurt sweetened with 15g (1 tbsp) honey. Use instead of the yoatie and assemble as above.

Balance Reduce the yoatie ingredient quantities to 130g (1½ cups) oats, 300ml (1¼ cups) apple juice and 90g (⅓ cup) yogurt.

First, make the yoatie. Mix the oats, apple juice and yogurt together in a bowl, then set aside in the fridge to soak for at least 2 hours (ideally, do this the day before).

Roughly crush the hazelnuts using a pestle and mortar or in a mug with the end of a rolling pin. Tip into a small microwaveable container along with the chocolate and melt on half-power at 15-second intervals until the chocolate has melted. Set aside and allow to cool.

Next, soak the gelatine in cold water for 10 minutes.

Meanwhile, put the apple juice, agave syrup and a few drops of peppermint extract, to taste, in a pan. Add the soaked gelatine and bring to the boil, stirring continuously.

Pour into a plastic container and place in the fridge and allow to set. (This will take a few hours so can also be done the day before). When the jelly is set, turn it out onto a board and cut into small cubes.

To serve, split the yoatie between 2 dessert bowls or large tumblers. Break up the nut and chocolate mixture into small pieces and sprinkle half on top of each along with 20g (¾oz) of the peppermint jelly cubes.

Mulled wine and mince pie yoatie

Transform the traditional indulgent mince pie into a 'good for you' favourite. You will find this yoatie is just too delicious to save for Christmas!

Health Another dish that is packed to the brim with antioxidants thanks to the purple grape juice.

Sport A superb breakfast that can be eaten cold, so pop in an airtight container and take to the gym for a quick morning fix after a workout.

SERVES 2

50g (⅓ cup) raisins

50g (1¾oz) mixed fruit peel

180g (2 cups) rolled oats

320ml (scant 1½ cups) purple grape juice

140g (⅔ cup) low-fat yogurt

finely grated zest of ½ orange

1 tsp in total of ground cinnamon, nutmeg and allspice

Reserve a handful of raisins and mixed peel. Then, mix the rest of the ingredients together in a bowl and leave in the fridge for at least 2 hours, or even overnight. Top with raisins and mixed fruit peel to serve.

Burn Replace the oats, purple grape juice and yogurt with 150g (⅔ cup) low-fat Greek yogurt sweetened with 15g (1 tbsp) honey. Mix the yogurt with the spices and fruit peel, top with a 30g (1¾oz) portion of black or red grapes and serve cold.

Balance Reduce the yoatie quantities to 140g (1⅔ cups) oats, 250ml (1 cup) purple grape juice and 110g (scant ½ cup) low-fat yogurt.

'Cherry Bakewell' yoatie

'After Eight' yoatie

Mulled wine and mince pie yoatie

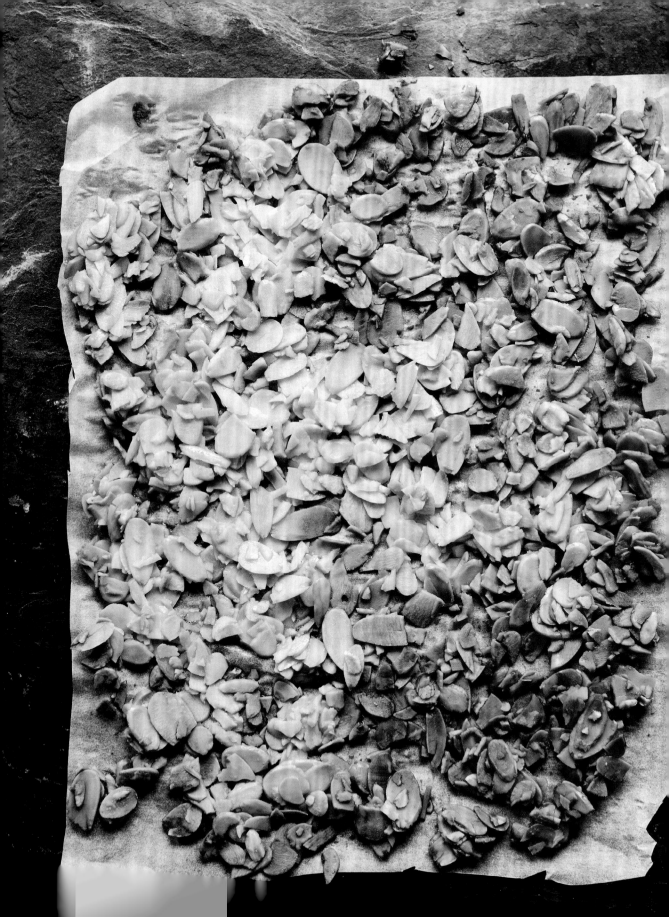

'Cherry Bakewell' yoatie

If there was ever a time to jazz up your oats, it's right now. Cherry and almond is a heavenly combination; if you like Bakewell tart then you will love this yoatie.

Health The high vitamin C content in this yoatie helps maintain immunity.

Sport The Montmorency cherries in the CherryActive have been shown to reduce muscle soreness following heavy exercise.

SERVES 2

FOR THE YOATIE:

185g (2¼ cups) rolled oats

280ml (1¼ cups) apple juice

130g (½ cup) natural yogurt

FOR THE JELLY (SERVES 8):

½ leaf gelatine

40g (1½oz) Morello cherries, pitted

40ml (1½ tbsp) CherryActive or apple juice

20g (3 tsp) agave syrup

FOR THE BRITTLE:

25g (3½ tsp) agave syrup

25g (1oz) egg white

100g (1 cup) flaked (slivered) almonds

First, make the yoatie. Mix the oats, apple juice and yogurt together in a bowl, then set aside in the fridge to soak for at least 2 hours (ideally, do this the day before).

Then, get on with the jelly. Soak the gelatine in cold water for 10 minutes. Put the cherries, CherryActive and agave syrup in a beaker and blitz until smooth using a hand-held blender.

Pour the purée into a pan and add the soaked gelatine and bring to the boil, stirring continuously. Pour into a cup or ramekin and place in the fridge and allow to set. (This will take a few hours, so can also be done the day before).

Preheat the oven to 160°C/325°F/gas mark 2½ and line a baking tray (cookie sheet) or a tray with baking parchment.

Lastly, for the brittle. Thoroughly mix the agave syrup and egg white together, stir in the almonds and spread out on the prepared tray, using a spatula to smooth it out into a thin layer. Bake in a preheated oven for 15 minutes until golden – the almonds should be stuck together and not wet when it's done. Remove from the oven and allow to cool.

To serve, split the yoatie between 2 dessert bowls or large tumblers. Use a fork to stir the cherry jelly until it's a smooth gel and then swirl through the yoatie. Break the almond brittle into small pieces and sprinkle 20g (¾oz) on top of each bowl.

Burn Replace the oats, apple juice and yogurt ingredients with 150g (⅔ cup) low-fat Greek yogurt sweetened with 15g (1 tbsp) honey. Use this mixture to replace the yoatie, and assemble as above.

Balance Reduce the quantity of yoatie ingredients to 130g (1½ cups) oats, 200ml (scant 1 cup) apple juice and 90g (⅓ cup) yogurt.

Apple crumble porridge

Apple and spice and all things nice! Nothing gives our insides a big warm hug more than yummy apple crumble. This scrumptious, gooey bowl of porridge (oatmeal) is all you need on a frosty morning.

Health A lactose- and gluten-free breakfast makes this perfect for those who have intolerances.

Sport Made with hazelnut milk to help give a deeper flavour, this porridge (oatmeal) is the tastiest carb-crammed kick start to your day.

SERVES 2

2 apples (we use Granny Smiths)

80g (1 cup) rolled oats

550ml (scant 2½ cups) hazelnut milk

¼ tsp ground cinnamon

¼ tsp ground nutmeg

40g (¼ cup) raisins

30g (1oz) granola (see page 71)

Peel and core the apples then dice them into small cubes (0.5cm/¼in).

In a hot non-stick frying pan (skillet) cook the cubed apple for 3–4 minutes until coloured all over.

Put the oats, hazelnut milk and spices into a non-stick pan and bring to the boil, reduce to a simmer and cook for a further 3–4 minutes.

To serve, divide the porridge (oatmeal) between 2 bowls and top with apple pieces, raisins and the granola. If eating solo, keep the rest of the porridge (oatmeal) in the fridge overnight and reheat, adding a little more milk, in the microwave on full power for 1–1½ minutes the next day.

Burn Replace the oats and hazelnut milk with 150g (⅔ cup) Greek yogurt sweetened with 15g (1 tbsp) honey. Mix the yogurt with the spices and raisins, serve cold and top with apple and granola.

Build Increase the quantities of oats to 50g (½ cup) and the hazelnut milk to 330ml (1½ cups) per portion.

DIY hazelnut milk

200g (1⅓ cups) unblanched hazelnuts
1 litre (4 cups) water
Place the nuts in a bowl and cover with water and leave overnight. Next, drain the water and empty the nuts into a jug blender. Add the water and blitz for 3–4 minutes.
Wet a piece of muslin cloth (cheesecloth) and wring the water out (the wet cloth works a lot better as it aids filtration). Fold it in half (to double up the layers) over a sieve (strainer) and strain the liquid into a bowl. When filtered, take the corners of the cloth and squeeze as much excess liquid out as possible. Serve the milk or keep in a sealed container in the fridge, where it will last for 3 days. You can dry the hazelnut pulp out on a baking tray (cookie sheet) in your oven, on its lowest setting; use it for baking in bars and breakfast toppings.

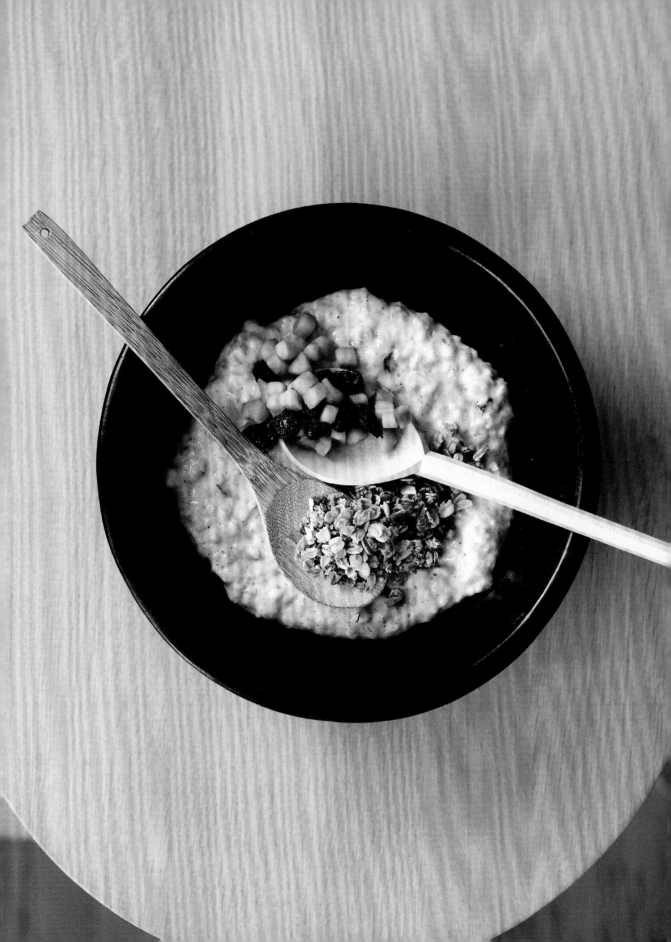

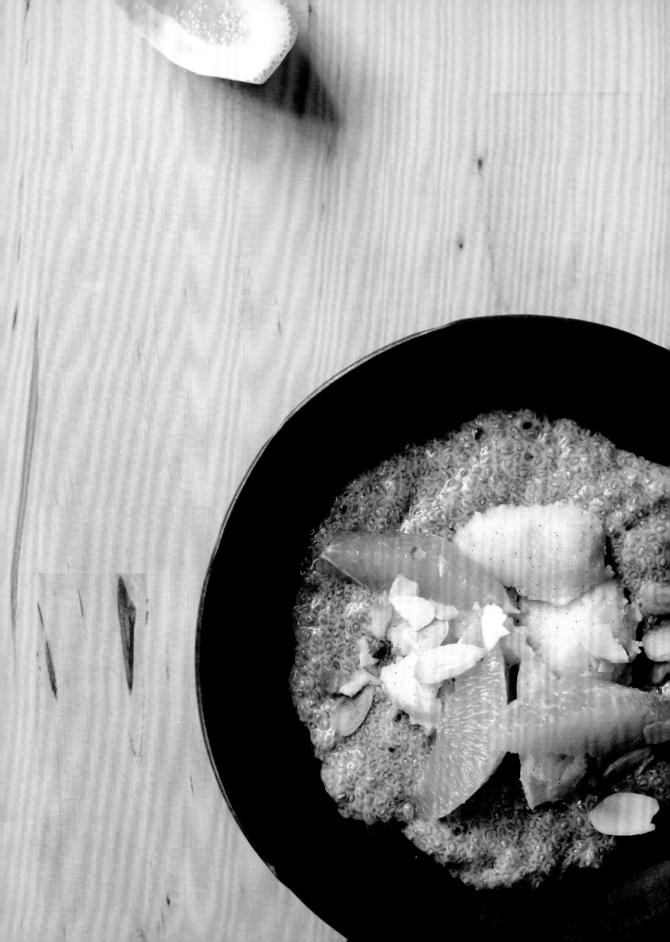

Semolina and chia porridge with orange, lemon and ginger

A breakfast with a great combination of textures and flavours, that's well worth the little extra effort. Once you've tried our flavour combo, then experiment with toppings of your favourite fruits and a handful of nuts.

Health Chia seeds are great for endurance sports as they form a gel in the stomach, which slows digestion and provides a slow release of carb fuel.

Sport The use of semolina helps improve cognitive brain function by being a great source of a number of B vitamins.

SERVES 2

FOR THE SEMOLINA:

35g (scant ¼ cup) semolina

20g (3 tsp) agave syrup

250ml (1 cup) semi-skimmed (lowfat) milk

juice of ½ lemon

finely grated zest of ¼ lemon

seeds from 1 vanilla pod (bean)

FOR THE CHIA PORRIDGE:

45g (¼ cup) chia seeds

180ml (generous ¾ cup) almond milk

½ tsp root ginger, finely chopped

30g (2 tbsp) honey

TO SERVE:

20g (¼ cup) flaked (slivered) almonds, toasted

1 orange, segmented

Place all the ingredients for the semolina into a pan and bring to the boil. Reduce to a simmer and cook for a further 3–4 minutes. Allow to cool and then chill in the fridge.

Next, make the chia porridge. Mix all the ingredients in a bowl and chill in the fridge for at least 1 hour.

To serve, spoon half of the chia porridge into each bowl, divide the set semolina between the bowls and top with half of the toasted almonds followed by the orange segments.

Burn Replace the semolina and milk with 125g (½ cup) low-fat Greek yogurt. Mix the rest of the ingredients for the semolina with the yogurt and serve on top of the chia porridge.

Build Double up the serving size of semolina.

Lychee, ginger and lemon quinoa porridge

Porridge (oatmeal) but with a lighter twist! Swapping the rolled oats for quinoa gives the dish a new, interesting dimension, that you may not have thought of trying before.

Health A very low-GI way to start your day: the slow-release carbs in the quinoa will keep your blood sugar levels stable throughout the morning, reducing urges to snack.

Top tip For a super-fast breakfast, make up a batch of this porridge but stop before you mix in the lychee and chill. Add the lychee and reheat in a microwave for 1–1½ minutes.

SERVES 2

20g (¾oz) stem (preserved) ginger, drained
350ml (1½ cups) apple juice
juice of ½ lemon
finely grated zest of 1 lemon
6 lychees
35g (¼ cup) quinoa

▽ **Burn** Replace the quinoa and the apple juice with 150g (⅔ cup) low-fat Greek yogurt with 15g (1 tbsp) honey. Mix in the rest of the ingredients and serve cold.

△ **Build** Increase the portion sizes by 25g (⅛ cup) quinoa and 250ml (1 cup) apple juice.

Blitz the ginger and apple juice in a blender or food processor, until the ginger is completely broken down. Then, add the lemon juice and zest.

Peel and stone the lychees and chop into small pieces.

Put the quinoa into a pan and pour over the apple juice mix. Cover with a lid and bring to the boil. Then, turn down and simmer until the juice has evaporated (just as if you were cooking rice) – about 20 minutes. Add a little more apple juice, if necessary – the quinoa should be quite light and fluffy.

Fold the lychees into the porridge and serve straightaway.

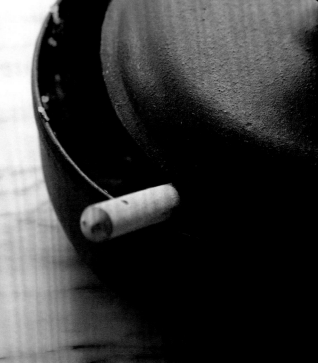
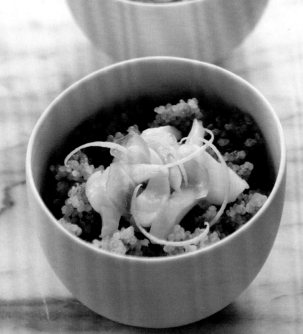

Coconut pancakes with papaya and macadamia butter

Pancakes are usually thought of as having very little nutritional merit, but with this specially designed – and gluten-free – recipe you can indulge yourself as each pancake contains less than 4g of carbohydrates.

Health Macadamia nuts are a good source of monounsaturated fats and are low in saturated fats – a great nutritional alternative to butter.

Top Tip Coconut flour contains nearly double the amount of protein found in wheat flour. It also provides instant energy, so it's great first thing.

MAKES 4/SERVES 2

FOR THE PAPAYA COMPÔTE:

1 large papaya, halved, deseeded and cut into cubes

2 tsp agave syrup

FOR THE NUT BUTTER:

100g (⅔ cup) macadamia nuts

30g (2 tbsp) salted butter, soft

FOR THE PANCAKES:

270ml (scant 1¼ cups) skimmed milk

¼ tsp xanthan gum

100g (scant 1 cup) coconut flour

3 large eggs

50ml (scant ¼ cup) coconut milk

1 tsp gluten-free baking powder

2 tsp vegetable oil, for frying

Balance Use 3 pancakes per portion.

Build In this variation you can have 4 pancakes per portion.

Put the cubed papaya and the agave syrup in a small pan and cook for 3–4 minutes over a medium heat until broken down. Transfer to a jar and allow to cool; keep this compôte in the fridge for up to 3 days.

Use a hand-held blender and a beaker to blitz the nuts and butter together. This nut butter can be stored in a jar in the fridge for up to 2 weeks.

Next, again using a hand-held blender and a beaker, blitz 120ml (½ cup) of the milk with the xanthan gum – what you want is something quite light and fluffy.

In a large bowl, put the coconut flour, eggs, coconut milk, baking powder and the rest of the milk. Mix well then fold in the milk–xanthan mixture.

Preheat a non-stick frying pan (skillet) over a low heat. Add 1 teaspoon of the oil and smear around the pan using some kitchen paper (paper towels). Add 1 tablespoon of the batter (or 2 separate tablespoons if your pan is big enough) to the pan and spread a little with the back of a spoon to about 8cm/3¼in. Cook for 2–3 minutes on each side; be gentle when flipping them over. These pancakes take a little longer than normal pancakes to cook, so the heat needs to be a touch lower so they don't colour too quickly. Add the rest of the oil after you have cooked half of the pancakes. These pancakes are best served warm, so as you'll be making batches keep them in a warm oven as you go. To serve a portion, stack 2 pancakes on a plate with half the papaya compôte. and top with a quenelle of nut butter, or layer up if you like.

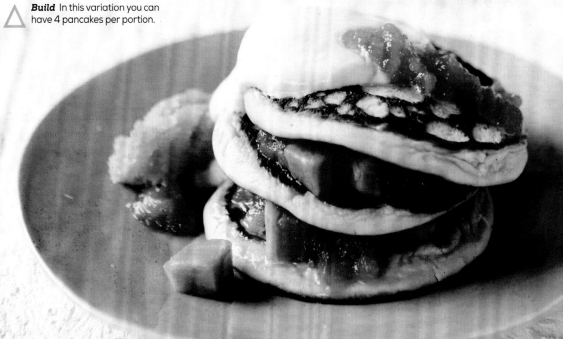

Two routes to a perfect pancake

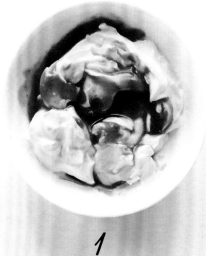

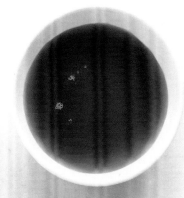

1

Strawberries, banana and cream

2

Turkey bacon and maple syrup

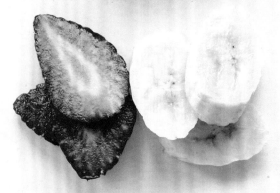

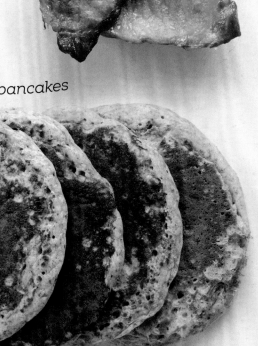

Heap onto pancakes

American pancakes, your way

The sweet aroma of coconut oil, warm pancake batter and delicious toppings will make your mind melt into a fluffy pancake heaven – we think this breakfast is less 'cheat' and more 'eat'.

Health By using buckwheat flour, these pancakes are high in fibre, manganese and magnesium. And they're gluten free too.

Sport The high protein content of these pancakes makes them ideal for kick starting muscle synthesis in the morning or as a post-training fix.

SERVES 2

FOR THE STRAWBERRY CREAM CHEESE:

50g (⅓ cup) strawberries

15g (1 tbsp) honey

60g (¼ cup) Greek yogurt

60g (¼ cup) low-fat cream cheese

FOR THE COMPÔTE:

170g (generous 1 cup) strawberries

20g (3 tsp) agave syrup

FOR THE TOPPINGS:

6 rashers (slices) turkey bacon

60g (scant ¼ cup) maple syrup

strawberries, halved, to serve

1 banana, sliced to serve

FOR THE PANCAKES:

100g (generous ¾ cup) buckwheat flour

20g (¾oz) unflavoured whey protein

1 tsp gluten-free baking powder

180ml (generous ¾ cup) skimmed milk

70g (⅓ cup) low-fat yogurt

20g (1 tbsp) honey

2 large eggs

coconut oil, for frying

First, make the strawberry cream cheese. Using a beaker and hand-held blender, blitz the strawberries with the honey and Greek yogurt. Then, add the cream cheese and mix thoroughly with a spoon and chill.

For the compôte, crush the strawberries with the back of a fork and place in a pan with the agave syrup. Bring to the boil over a medium heat, stirring continuously until it starts to thicken, about 2–3 minutes. When done, transfer to a small container and refrigerate.

Preheat the oven to 110°C/225°F/gas mark ¼ and the grill (broiler) to medium hot. Grill (broil) the turkey bacon for 2–3 minutes on each side, then keep warm, wrapped in foil to stop it drying out, in a low oven.

Sift the flour, protein and baking powders into a large bowl. In a separate bowl or jug (pitcher), whisk together the milk, yogurt, honey and eggs. Pour the liquid mixture into the flour mixture and, using a whisk, beat until you have a smooth batter. Let stand for a few minutes.

Next, heat a non-stick frying pan (skillet) over a medium heat and add ½ teaspoon of coconut oil and smear about when melted using a folded piece of kitchen paper (paper towel) – you don't want an oily pan, just a thin coating of oil. Repeat this oiling after every two or three pancakes. Pour or ladle the batter into the pan until it spreads to 10cm (4in) in diameter (do 2 at a time if your pan is big enough). It might seem very thick but this is how it should be. Wait until the top of the pancake begins to bubble, then turn it over and cook until both sides are golden brown and the pancake has risen to about 1cm (½in) high. Repeat until all the batter is used up; keep the cooked pancakes warm in a low oven.

Serve 3 pancakes per portion along with half of the strawberry cream cheese, a swirl of compôte and half the sliced banana or serve with the maple syrup and bacon – whichever you prefer. If you're eating solo, then you can cook all the pancakes and once cool store them in an airtight container in the fridge for 2–3 days or freeze them. You can reheat them in the oven (160°C/325°F/gas mark 2½) for 3–4 minutes from chilled and for 6–8 minutes from frozen.

Burn Use the coconut pancakes (see page 81), instead.

Build Increase the portion size to 4 pancakes.

Bacon, hash brown and egg with 'cheese on toast' sauce

Who says you can't eat a great-tasting cooked breakfast that's good for you too? Here's the proof – and once you've made this amazing 'cheese on toast' sauce, you'll be wanting to eat it every day.

Health Tomatoes are rich in antioxidants and lycopene; research shows that both are important for bone health. If you're doing lots of high-impact activity, be sure to snack on tomatoes and benefit your bones at the same time.

Top tip Seek out orange- and tangerine-coloured tomatoes as they contain a type of lycopene that's more easily absorbed than that in their red cousins.

SERVES 2

50g (1¾oz) medium Cheddar

1 slice wholemeal (wholewheat) bread

300g (10½oz) potato (we use Maris Piper), peeled

2 tsp plain (all-purpose) flour

a pinch of salt

1 tsp vegetable oil

4 rashers (slices) back (Canadian) bacon

120g (4½oz) cherry tomatoes

2 tbsp white wine vinegar

2 large eggs

150ml (⅔ cup) semi-skimmed (lowfat) milk

40g (1½oz) spinach leaves

Burn Replace the hash brown with a grilled (broiled) flat mushroom and 2 spears of grilled (broiled) asparagus per portion.

Build Add a portion of granary toast or a serving of baked beans (see page 86) to your breakfast.

Preheat the oven to 160°C/325°F/gas mark 2½, and line 2 baking trays (cookie sheets) with baking parchment.

Grate the Cheddar onto 1 of the prepared baking trays (cookie sheets) and place in a preheated oven until golden brown all over (about 8–10 minutes). At the same time place the slice of bread onto another baking tray (cookie sheet), place in the oven until lightly browned all over, remove and set aside. Then, turn up the oven temperature to 180°C/350°F/gas mark 4.

Bring a large pan of water to the boil and add the potato (you're going to use this pan and water for the poached eggs, too, so it should be as deep as possible). Cook for 10 minutes and then lift out of the water.

Using a tea (dish) towel to hold the potato, grate it into a bowl then add the flour and salt and mix in well. Halve the mixture and press each half into a large pastry cutter to form a round patty. Transfer the patties to a hot non-stick frying pan (skillet) over a medium heat with the oil. Cook until golden brown on both sides, transfer to a prepared tray and cook in the oven for 15–20 minutes.

Trim the bacon of excess fat and cook on a baking tray (cookie sheet) until your liking. Cook the tomatoes at the same time for 8–10 minutes.

Add the vinegar to the pan of water and bring back to the boil, reduce the heat to a simmer and crack the eggs into the water. Cook for 3 minutes and then remove using a large slotted spoon.

Meanwhile, in a small pan bring the milk to the boil then remove from the heat. Remove the cheese from the baking tray and put into a blender with half of the toast, blitz and slowly pour in the milk; you might need to add more pieces of toast to achieve a sauce consistency. Add salt to taste.

Finally, wilt the spinach in a non-stick frying pan (skillet) over a medium heat and serve straightaway. We like to plate the spinach and tomatoes together then stack the hash brown, bacon and egg on top and pour over the sauce.

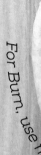

For Burn, use mushroom

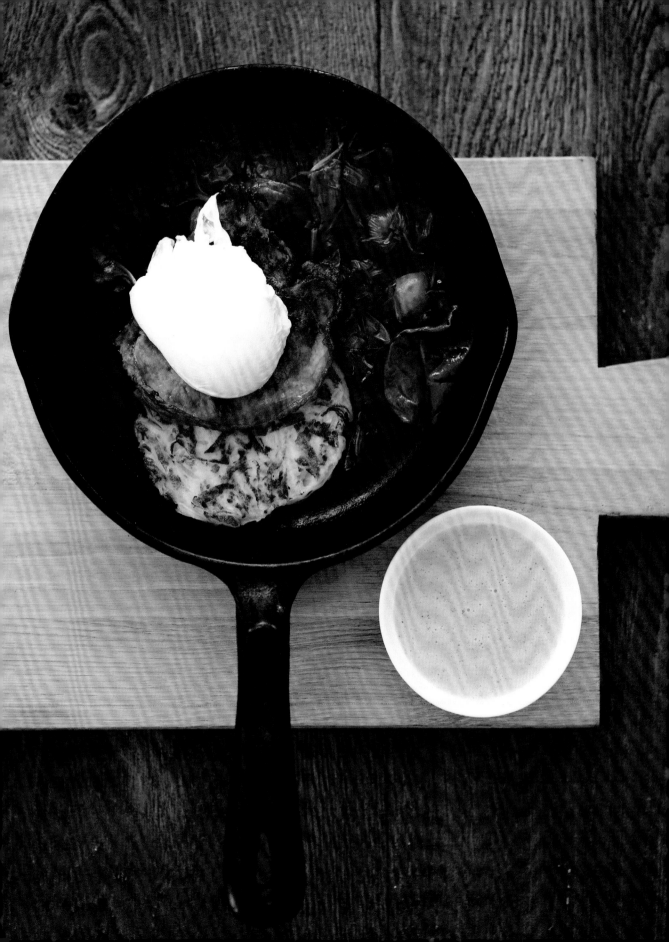

Healthy English breakfast

A guilt-free alternative to the Sunday morning, greasy fry-up. By tweaking cooking methods and sourcing fresh lean ingredients you can still enjoy the traditional full English classic and it will put you a step closer to your goal rather than two steps back.

Top tip If you like, you can also make your own ketchup – one not filled with preservatives, salt and sugar (home-made is the real thing) – simply use the tomato sauce recipe below (or the one on page 89) and store in a jam jar in the fridge for use later on.

Sport This full English provides a great hit of protein to fuel protein synthesis first thing of a morning.

SERVES 2

120g (¾ cup) cooked cannellini beans, drained and rinsed

2 reduced-fat sausages

2 rashers (slices) back (Canadian) bacon

2 forestière or large flat mushrooms

3 eggs

40ml (1½ tbsp) semi-skimmed (lowfat) milk

sea salt and freshly ground black pepper, to taste

FOR THE TOMATO SAUCE (SERVES 4):

½ onion, finely diced

½ clove garlic, roughly chopped or crushed

1 tsp vegetable oil

400g (14oz) tin chopped tomatoes

2 tbsp tomato purée (paste)

1 sprig fresh thyme, leaves picked

First, make the tomato sauce for the baked beans. Place the onion and garlic in a medium-sized pan with the oil, on a medium heat, and cook until soft (you don't want any colour on them).

Next add the tomatoes and tomato purée (paste) and bring to a simmer. Continue to cook until it has reduced by a third. Meanwhile, preheat the oven to 180°C/350°F/gas mark 4.

Allow the tomato sauce to cool a little before pouring into a blender, then add the thyme leaves and blitz until smooth.

Place the beans in a pan with 100g/3½oz (or a quarter) of the tomato sauce and set aside. (If you prefer you can double up the beans and use all of the tomato sauce, or freeze the sauce for another time.)

Put the sausages and bacon on a baking tray (cookie sheet) and bake in the oven for 15–20 minutes (times will vary depending on how thick the sausage is and how crispy you like your bacon). At the same time, put the mushrooms in a small ovenproof dish and bake for 10–12 minutes. When they're done drain off any liquid into the pan of baked beans.

Meanwhile, reheat the beans on a low heat, stirring occasionally. When hot, taste and add a little salt, if necessary.

Next, whisk the eggs and the milk together in a bowl or jug (pitcher) and pour into a medium-sized non-stick pan. Cook on a medium heat, stirring all the time with a wooden spoon. When the eggs are nearly done fold in the spinach and add a little salt, to taste.

Divide the baked beans, bacon, sausages, mushrooms and scrambled egg between 2 plates and then season with black pepper (to taste) and serve straightaway.

Burn Remove the cannellini beans and add 60g (2¼oz) roasted tomatoes instead per portion.

Build Add one slice of wholemeal (wholewheat) or granary toast per portion.

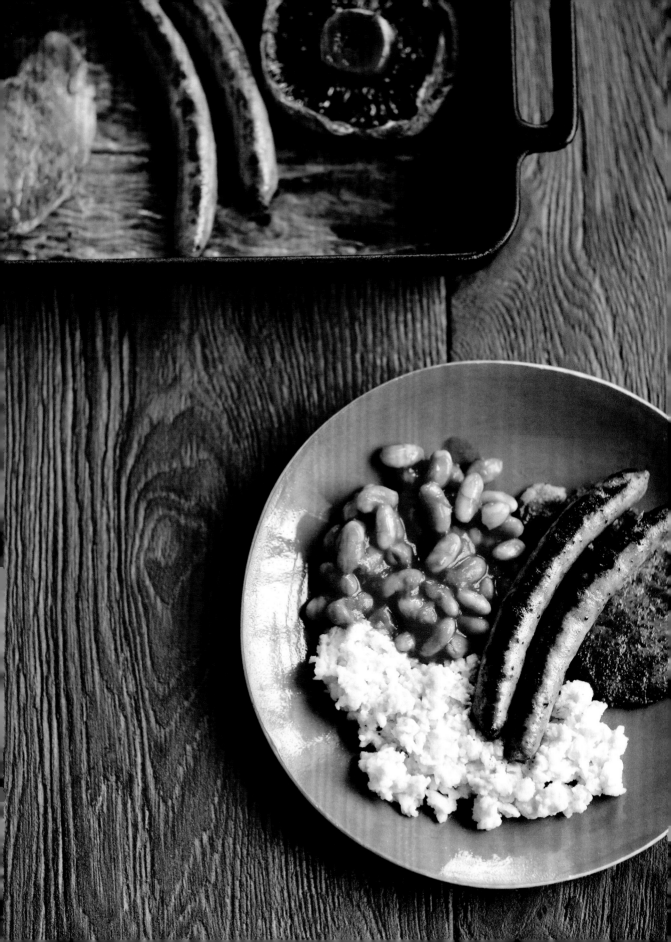

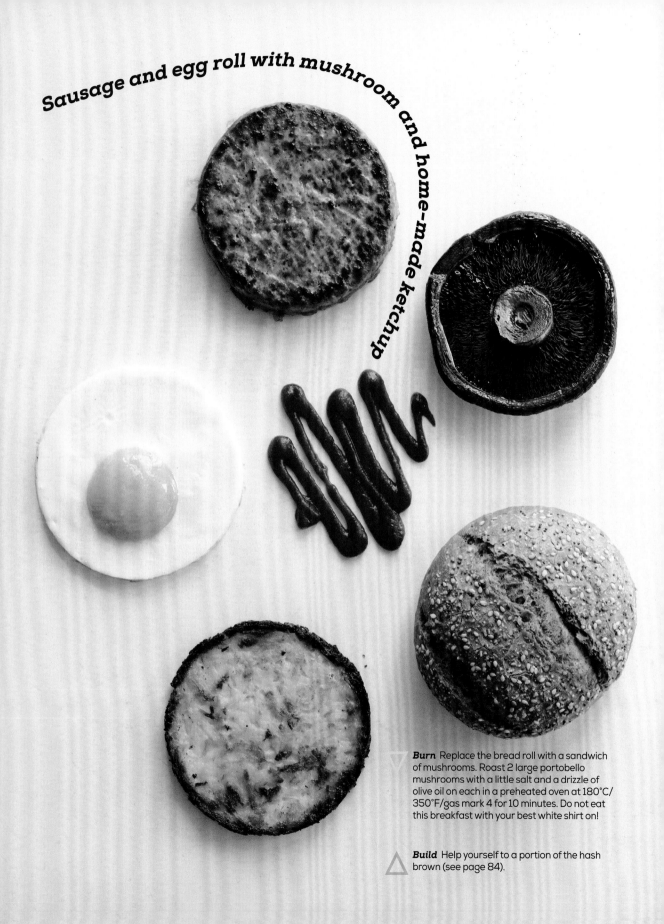

Sausage and egg roll with mushroom and home-made ketchup

Burn Replace the bread roll with a sandwich of mushrooms. Roast 2 large portobello mushrooms with a little salt and a drizzle of olive oil on each in a preheated oven at 180°C/350°F/gas mark 4 for 10 minutes. Do not eat this breakfast with your best white shirt on!

Build Help yourself to a portion of the hash brown (see page 84).

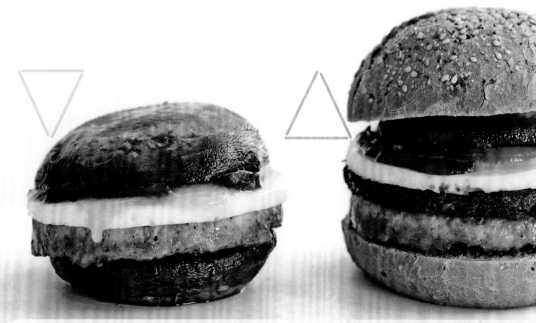

Usually reserved for 'greasy spoon' cafés or fast-food outlets, this take on the sausage and egg muffin is perfect for a Sunday morning 'treat' without the guilt.

Health This roll is bursting with micronutrients and has none of the trans fats or artificial ingredients of the fast-food version.

Top tip Because you're mostly eating healthy and nutritious foods, you can eat this without tipping the scales nutritionally.

SERVES 2

2 portobello mushrooms

2 large eggs

2 wholemeal (wholewheat) or granary rolls

2 tsp spreadable light butter

FOR THE KETCHUP:

400g (14oz) tin chopped tomatoes

½ onion, diced

1 clove garlic, crushed

30g (1oz) sundried tomato

¼ tsp allspice

3 tsp agave syrup

4 tsp white wine vinegar

FOR THE SAUSAGE PATTIES:

1 tsp sea salt

¼ tsp ground mace

¼ tsp ground cloves

1 tsp ground black pepper

2 tsp chopped sage leaves

500g (1lb 2oz) extra-lean pork mince (ground pork)

2 tsp vegetable oil, for frying

First, make the ketchup by putting all of the ingredients apart from the vinegar into a pan. Bring to the boil, reduce to a simmer and continue to cook for 20 minutes. Remove from the heat and allow to cool a little. Transfer the pan's contents to a jug blender and blitz for 5–10 minutes – you want the sauce to be super-smooth. Return the sauce to the pan and reduce over a medium heat to create a thick consistency. Add the vinegar for the last few minutes of cooking time. Allow the sauce to cool. Store in an airtight container or jar in the fridge for up to 2 weeks.

Preheat the oven to 180°C/350°F/gas mark 4, and line a baking tray (cookie sheet) with baking parchment. Now, make the sausage patties. Grind the salt, spices and herbs (in a pestle and mortar, hand-held blender with beaker or spice mill). Tip into a bowl with the pork and mix.

Divide the mixture into 4 and press each into a 10cm (4in) cutter or ring to form a patty. Add 1 teaspoon of the oil to a hot frying pan (skillet) and cook the desired amount of sausage patties for 2 minutes on each side (this recipe makes 4 patties, so keep any remaining patties in the fridge for up to 3 days or freeze for use another day).

Remove the patties from the pan and transfer to the baking tray (cookie sheet) with the mushrooms and cook in the oven for 10–12 minutes.

Meanwhile, cook the eggs using the remaining oil in small blini pans or a larger non-stick frying pan (skillet). For a neat stack, crack the eggs into the cleaned 10cm (4in) rings you used to make the sausage patties. When the patties and eggs are done, slice the rolls and spread on the light butter. On the base of the roll, place a sausage patty followed by a mushroom, an egg and the desired amount of tomato ketchup. Close with the top half of the muffin and enjoy straightaway.

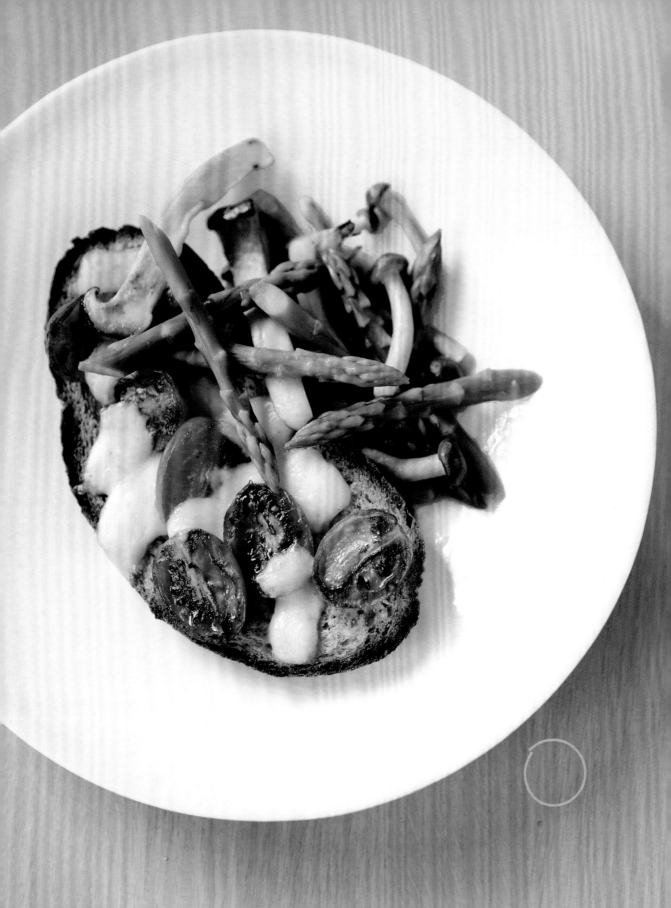

Wild mushrooms, asparagus, tomatoes and cheese on toast

Taking good old cheese on toast to new heights with earthy mushrooms, sweet tomatoes and succulent asparagus - with this breakfast, you can't go wrong.

Health This fibre-full breakfast will fill you up all morning, reducing the chance of you making unhealthy snack choices before lunchtime.

Sport This dish is a great source of vitamin K, found in the asparagus. Vitamin K is vital for blood clotting, wound healing and maintaining strong bones.

SERVES 2

100g (3½oz) baby plum tomatoes, halved

120g (4½oz) asparagus tips

2 slices wholemeal (wholewheat) or granary bread

60g (¼oz) low-fat mozzarella (about ½ ball), sliced or torn

1 tsp extra virgin olive oil

250g (9oz) mixed wild mushrooms (tear or slice large ones into smaller pieces)

Burn Replace the toast with a portion of scrambled egg made with 1 whole egg and 1 egg white; or have a boiled or poached egg if you prefer.

Build Serve with a portion of hash brown (see page 84).

Preheat the grill (broiler) to medium hot.

Meanwhile, place the tomato halves cut-side down in a hot non-stick frying pan (skillet) over a high heat. Cook until caramelised on this side.

Cook the asparagus tips in a pan of boiling water for 3 minutes.

Lightly toast the bread on both sides. Place on a baking tray (cookie sheet) and top each slice with the tomatoes and pieces of mozzarella. Place under the grill (broiler) until the cheese has melted.

Add the oil to the frying pan (skillet) and cook the mushrooms over a high heat for 2–3 minutes until browned slightly and softened.

Divide all the ingredients between 2 plates and serve.

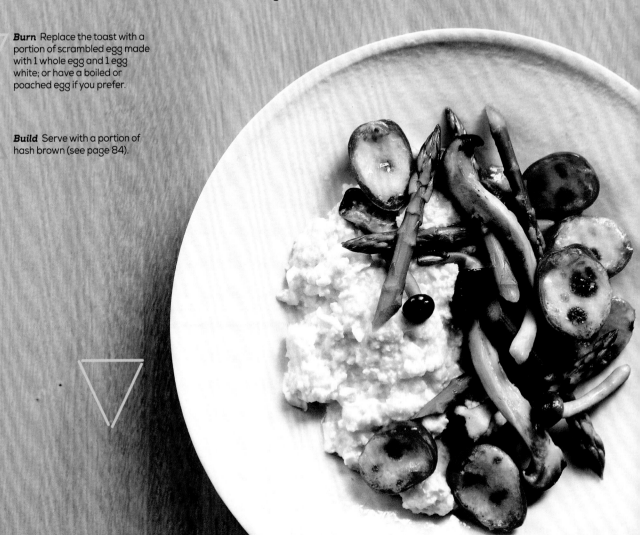

Soulmatefood-style smoked salmon and scrambled eggs

This super-healthy dish disguises itself under a layer of luxury and indulgence and delivers a perfectly balanced start to your day, including protein, complex carbs, healthy fats and antioxidants.

Health Smoked salmon, avocado and eggs are all packed full of healthy fats – monounsaturated fats (avocado) and omega-3s (salmon and eggs).

Sport Due to its anti-inflammatory properties, this dish is fantastic for any sports person who is trying to reduce inflammation and the risk of injury.

SERVES 2

150g (5½oz) cherry or baby plum tomatoes (mixed colour if possible), halved lengthways

1 avocado

juice of ½ lemon

160g (5¾oz) sliced cold-smoked salmon

4 slices rye bread

3 eggs

40g (1½ tbsp) semi-skimmed (lowfat) milk

1½ tsp chopped chives

salt and freshly ground black pepper, to taste

30g (2 tbsp) spreadable light butter

pumpkin seeds, to garnish (optional)

Preheat the oven to 80°C/176°F or whatever the lowest setting of your oven is, and you'll need a baking tray (cookie sheet).

Place the tomato halves cut-side down in an ovenproof, non-stick frying pan (skillet) or in a non-stick roasting tin over a high heat for 2–3 minutes until starting to caramelise. Then transfer to the oven.

Halve the avocado and remove the stone. Cut each half into 4 pieces lengthways and, using a knife, remove the skin. Squeeze over the lemon juice and place on a baking tray (cookie sheet) in the oven.

Lay the smoked salmon on a plate and place in the oven while you toast the bread and cook the eggs. Bear in mind that you only want the avocado and the salmon to be warm, you're not trying to cook them.

Whisk the eggs and the milk together in a bowl or jug (pitcher) and pour into a medium-sized non-stick pan. Cook on a medium heat and stir with a wooden spoon. When the eggs are nearly done sprinkle over the chives and a little salt, to taste.

When the toast is done, spread with the light butter and put 2 slices on each plate. Divide the salmon between the plates and share out the scrambled eggs, avocado and tomatoes and serve, with a few twists of black pepper and a few pumpkin seeds, if you like.

 Burn Remove the toast and replace with 2 spears of grilled (broiled) asparagus and 40g (1½oz) wilted spinach per portion.

 Build Add an extra slice of toast or replace the toast with a hot bagel along with 25g (scant ¼ cup) cream cheese.

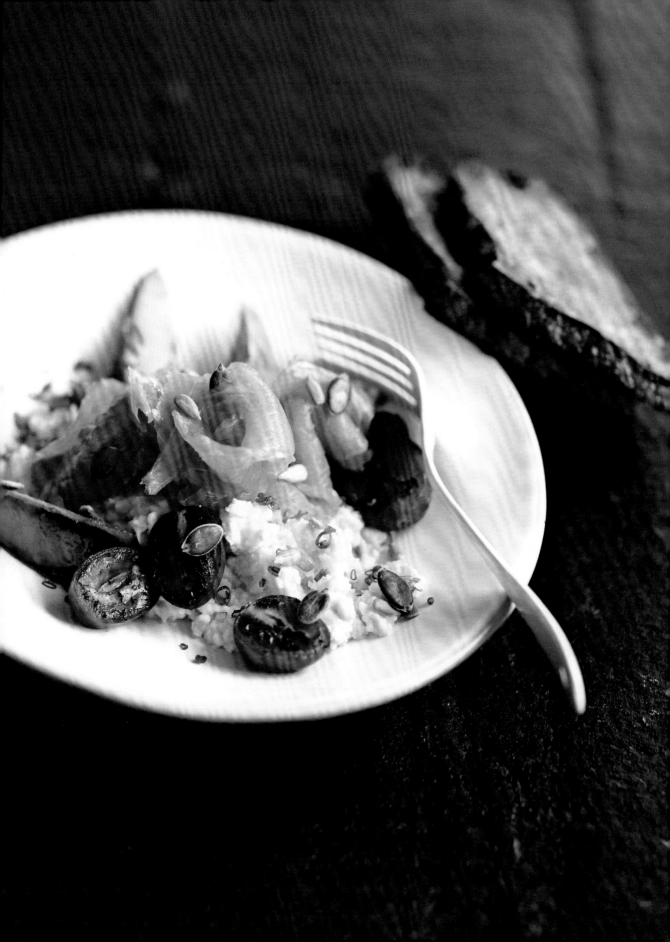

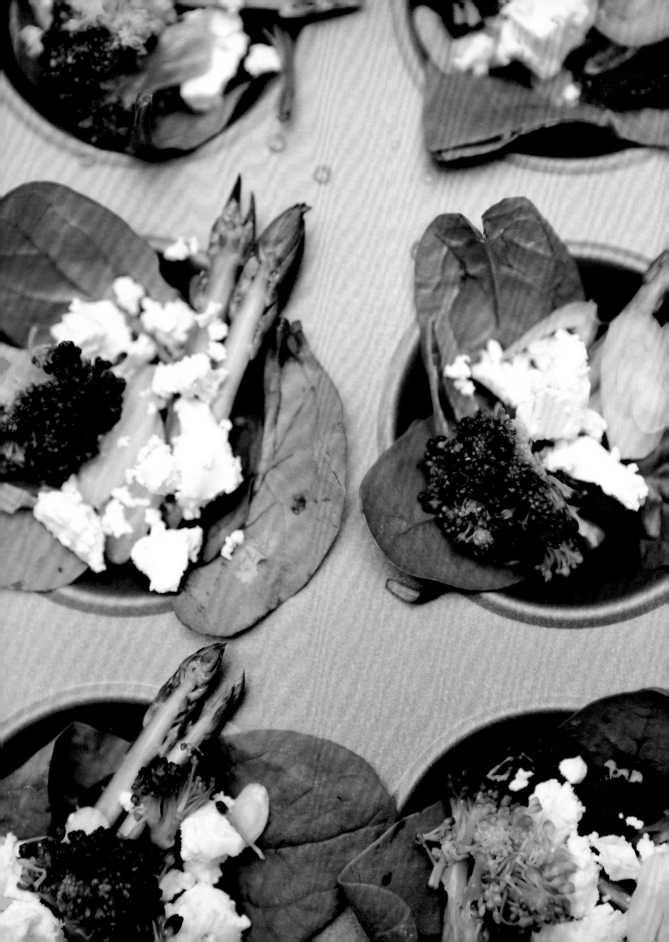

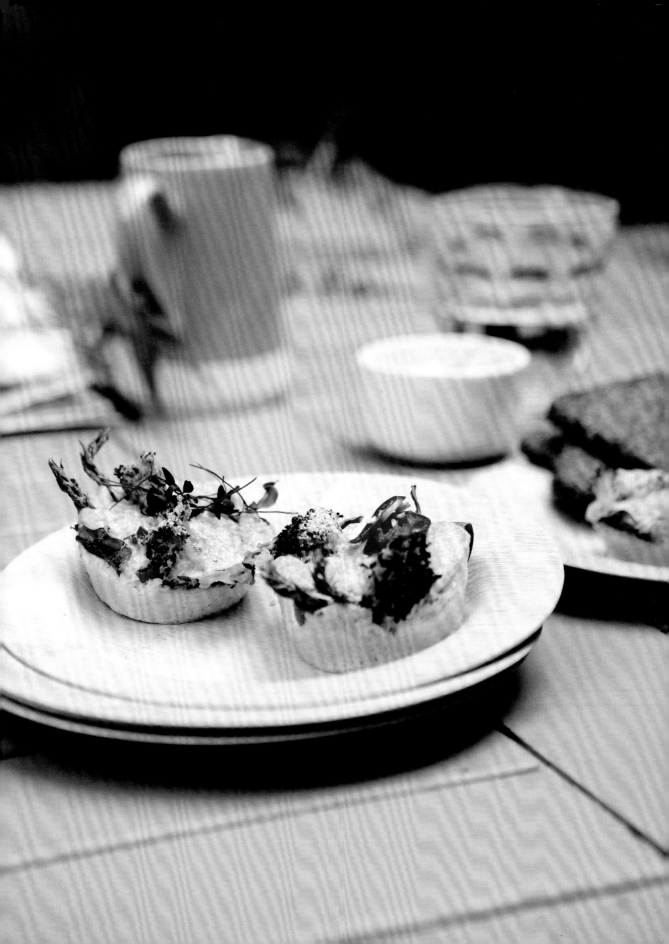

Broccoli, Peppadew and feta mini frittatas with asparagus

Start your day with a burst of colour and two of these delicious and filling frittatas for breakfast. Pop them in the oven before your morning shower and they'll be ready by the time you are.

Health These little frittatas are packed with both kinds of fibre (insoluble and soluble), which is great for keeping your digestive system in top working order.

Sport Being high in calcium, these frittatas can help to maintain bone health during high-impact endurance sports, such as marathon training.

MAKES 6

50g (1¾oz) broccoli, cut into florets
6 eggs
18 baby spinach leaves
50g (1¾oz) feta cheese
50g (1¾oz) asparagus
50g (1¾oz) Peppadew peppers, cut into quarters
5g (⅙oz) chives, chopped
micro basil, to garnish
1 slice of rye bread, to serve

Preheat the oven to 180°C/350°F/gas mark 4 and you'll also need a 6- or 12-hole non-stick muffin tin.

Cook the broccoli in boiling water for 3–4 minutes and then refresh in iced water to keep the colour and stop the cooking.

Separate the eggs, putting the whites in one bowl and the yolks in another. Whisk the whites until firm peaks form. Whisk the yolks until they've broken down. Then fold the egg whites into the yolks.

Line the muffin tin with 3 baby spinach leaves in each of 6 of the muffin tin holes. Crumble in the feta followed by the cooked broccoli.

Take the woody bottoms off the asparagus and slice up the rest, keeping the tips whole. Add the sliced asparagus to the frittatas, cut each asparagus tip in half and lean the two halves on the side of each hole.

Divide the Peppadew peppers and the chopped chives between the frittatas. Finally, add the egg mixture just to the top of the moulds and bake in a preheated oven for 12–15 minutes. To test if they're ready, insert the tip of a knife into the middle of the frittata, if it comes out clean then they're cooked, if not pop back in for a few more minutes.

When done, remove from the oven, allow to cool and remove from the tin. Garnish with micro basil and serve with a slice of rye bread.

These mini-breakfasts store well in an airtight container, but do eat them within 3 days. We don't think that'll be hard.

 Burn Follow the recipe above, omitting the rye bread to serve.

 Build Follow the recipe above and add an extra slice of rye bread per portion. If you've got any cooked sweet potato or similar left over from the night before, try adding 50g (1¾oz) of this to the frittata mix.

Banana and walnut bread with Earl Grey cream

This breakfast is one of our favourite foods in the Soulmatefood kitchen! It makes both a great satisfying start to the day or a lovely mid-morning snack – we like ours with a cup of green tea.

Health A good pre-gym booster that will deliver enough quick energy to get you through an early morning session without feeling too full.

Top tip You can freeze this gluten-free fruit bread in slices and pop it in the toaster for those mornings when time is tight.

SERVES 8

FOR THE BANANA AND WALNUT BREAD:

125g (9 tbsp) spreadable light butter

160g (¾ cup) soft brown sugar

2 large eggs

½ tsp vanilla extract

125g (1 cup) buckwheat flour

125g (¾ cup) brown rice flour

2 tsp gluten-free baking powder

3 ripe bananas

120g (1 cup) walnuts, chopped

FOR THE EARL GREY CREAM:

50ml (scant ¼ cup) semi-skimmed (lowfat) milk

2 Earl Grey tea bags

30g (1oz) unflavoured whey protein

110g (½ cup) quark or crème fraîche

25g (3½ tsp) agave syrup

Preheat the oven to 180°C/350°F/gas mark 4, and then line a 1lb loaf tin with baking parchment.

Cream together the light butter and the sugar until light and fluffy, using a free-standing mixer or electric hand mixer. Whisk in the eggs one at a time until mixed thoroughly and add the vanilla extract.

Put the flours and baking powder together in a bowl and fold this dry mixture into the eggy mix a third at a time until fully incorporated.

Crush the bananas with the back of a fork and fold into the mixture along with the walnuts.

Pour the mixture into the prepared tin and bake in a preheated oven for 45–50 minutes. Check that it's done by inserting a skewer into the middle of the loaf, it should come out clean. Allow the loaf to cool completely in the tin on a wire rack.

While the loaf is cooling, make the cream. Heat the milk with the tea bags in a small pan and bring to the boil. Remove from the heat and allow the Earl Grey flavours to infuse for 10 minutes. Remove the tea bags and discard, transfer the liquid into a beaker and allow to cool.

Once cool, mix in the rest of the ingredients to form a smooth, thick cream. Store this cream in an airtight container in the fridge for up to 3 days.

Cut 2 slices (1cm/½in thick) of the bread per portion and serve with 1 tablespoon of the fragrant tea cream.

Burn Serve a slice using the 80/20 rule (see page 10).

Balance Reduce the portion size to 1 slice.

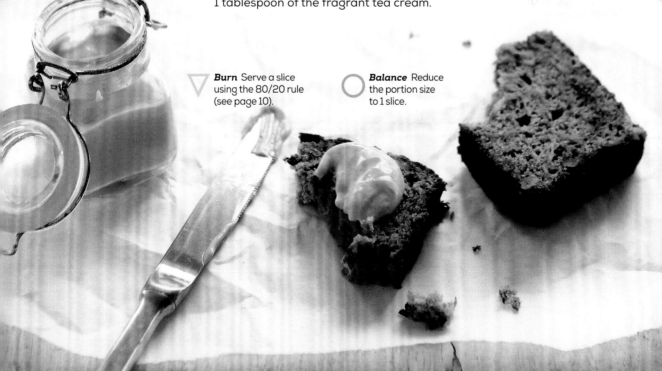

Corn cakes with goat's cheese and home-made baked beans

Ooh when it's chilly outside first thing, warm yourself up with these rustic corn cakes and tangy beans.

Health This breakfast is high in fibre to promote healthy bowel function.

Sport The beans are high in folate, which will help maintain your red blood cell count, helping to improve endurance levels and to reduce the risk of anaemia.

SERVES 2

FOR THE CORN CAKES:

spreadable light butter, for greasing

280g (10oz) cooked sweetcorn (tinned and drained or stripped off the cob)

2 eggs, separated

40g (⅓ cup) medium cornmeal or polenta

60g (scant ½ cup) plain (all-purpose) flour

½ tsp gluten-free baking powder

½ tsp salt

¼ tsp fine ground black pepper

4g (⅛oz) chives

100g (scant ½ cup) soft goat's cheese

FOR THE BAKED BEANS:

½ onion, finely diced

½ clove garlic, roughly chopped or crushed

1 tsp vegetable oil

400g (14oz) tin chopped tomatoes

10g (2 tsp) agave syrup

40g tomato purée (paste)

dried chilli (red pepper) flakes (optional)

240g (1⅔ cups) cooked pinto or borlotti beans (or a 410g/ 14oz tin, drained)

Preheat the oven to 170°C/344°F/gas mark 3 and lightly grease a shallow non-stick 6-hole Yorkshire pudding tin with light butter.

Set aside 70g (2½oz) of sweetcorn in a bowl, blitz the rest of the sweetcorn in a food processor (or use a hand-held blender) until broken down to a wet hummus-like texture, then transfer to a medium-sized bowl. Mix the egg yolks into the blitzed sweetcorn using a wooden spoon.

In a separate bowl, mix the cornmeal, flour, baking powder and seasoning together, and then add this dry mix to the sweetcorn mixture a third at a time. Finely chop the chives and crumble in the goat's cheese then stir both into the mix.

Whisk the egg whites with a balloon whisk or electric whisk until they form soft peaks and, using a wooden spoon or a spatula, gently fold the egg whites and the remaining sweetcorn into the mixture, being very careful not to overmix as you want the batter to be as light as possible.

Evenly divide the batter into each 'hole' of the tin, giving the tray a gentle tap to help it settle. Bake in the preheated oven for 15 minutes until the tops are just starting to turn colour. These are best served straight out of the oven but can be chilled and reheated later.

Now, make the baked beans. Place the onion and garlic in a medium-sized pan with the oil, on a medium heat, and cook until soft (you don't want any colour on them).

Next add the tomatoes, agave syrup, tomato purée (paste) and a few chilli (red pepper) flakes (if using) – just add a little at a time and let it cook out for a few minutes before you taste it; you can always add more, but can't take it away – then bring it to a simmer. Cook until it has reduced by a third. Allow to cool a little and transfer to a blender and blitz until smooth.

Rinse the beans in a sieve (strainer) under cold water and tip into a pan with 100g (3½oz) of the tomato sauce over a low heat, occasionally stirring. When the beans are hot add a little salt, if necessary, to taste.

To serve, place 3 corn cakes a piece on a plate with a heap of the home-made baked beans alongside.

Burn Reduce the portion size to 2 corn cakes, use this breakfast under the 80/20 rule (see page 10).

Build Give yourself 2 slices of grilled (broiled) bacon as an extra side.

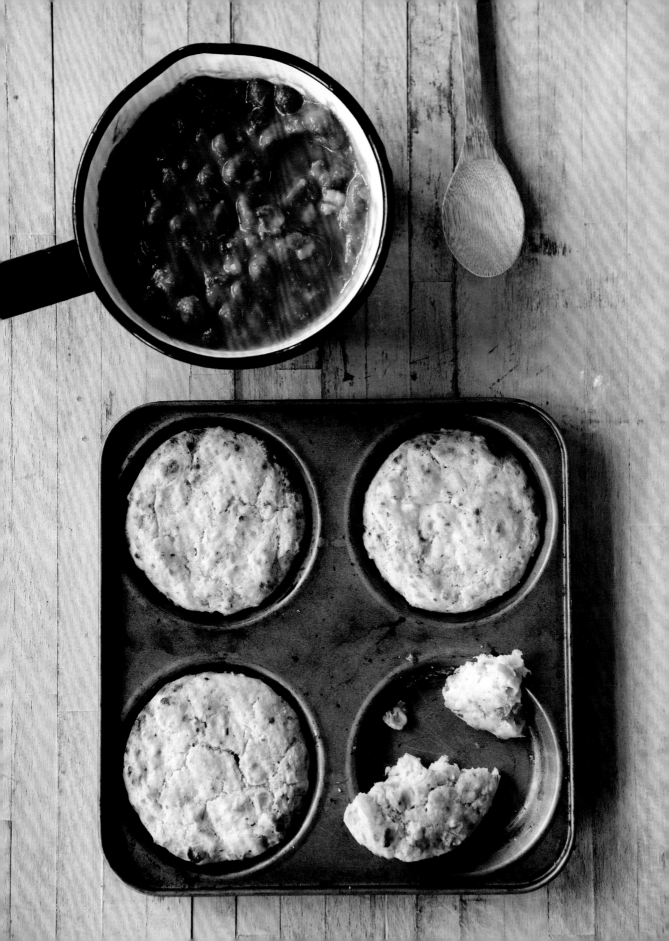

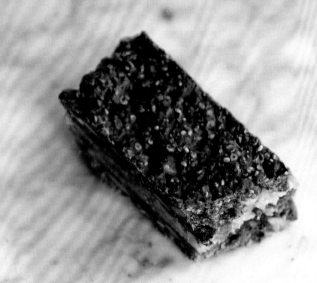

SoulSaver breakfast bar

If you are guilty of skipping breakfast or grabbing a processed and highly sugared breakfast bar then stop right there! This breakfast bar is the only one you'll ever need. It covers all the bases nutritionally, so there's no need to grab and go with anything else.

Health A complete bar – it contains low-GI carbs, healthy fats and protein, plus a great source of many micronutrients vital for a productive day.

Top tip For variety try including a few drops of your favourite flavoured essence or essential oil – we've found peppermint or orange-flower water both work well.

MAKES 6

25g (scant ¼ cup) chia seeds
45g (1½ tbsp) apple juice
100g coconut oil
100g (½ cup) agave syrup
30g (⅓ cup) porridge (rolled) oats
90g (½ cup) quinoa flakes
35g (¼ cup) hazelnuts, chopped
25g (¼ cup) goji berries
25g (¼ cup) sunflower seeds
35g (1¼oz) unflavoured whey protein
3 tsp spirulina
1 tsp finely chopped root ginger
2 tsp cocoa powder
½ tsp ground cinnamon

▽ **Burn** Divide the loaf into 8 portions.

△ **Build** Divide the loaf into 5 portions.

Preheat the oven to 170°C/344°F/gas mark 3, and then line a 1lb loaf tin with baking parchment.

Soak the chia seeds in the apple juice in a cup or small bowl for 1 hour.

In a small pan melt the coconut oil and the agave syrup together.

Using a free-standing mixer, or in a large bowl with a wooden spoon, mix the oats, quinoa, hazelnuts, goji berries, sunflower seeds and protein. Then tip in the coconut agave mixture along with the soaked chia and any remaining juice. Using a paddle beater, or a wooden spoon, mix everything together thoroughly. Divide this mixture into thirds.

Put one-third into the prepared loaf tin and press down firmly.

Mix another third with the spirulina and ginger, then on a chopping (cutting) board press this into the rough shape and size of the bottom of the loaf tin. Transfer this third to the loaf tin and sit it on top of the first layer, pressing down with a spatula to fill the space, as necessary.

With the last third, mix in the cocoa and cinnamon and repeat as before to form a third layer and top the loaf tin. Cover with foil and bake in a preheated oven for 25 minutes. Remove from the oven and allow to cool in the tin before slicing into portions. One portion is one-sixth of the loaf, so slice into 6 and store in an airtight container, where these bars will last for 5 days.

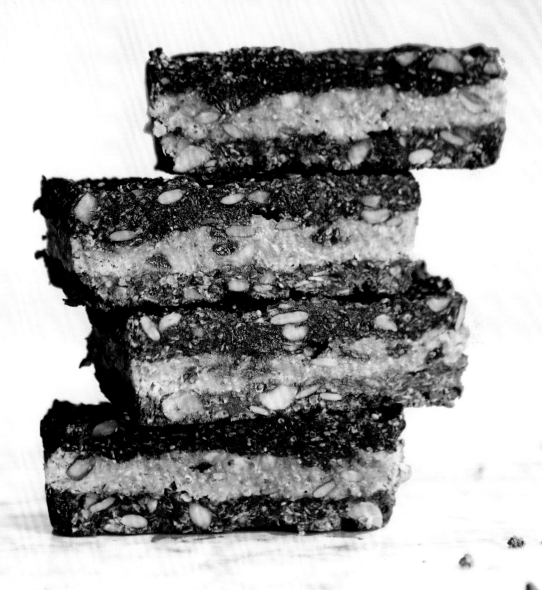

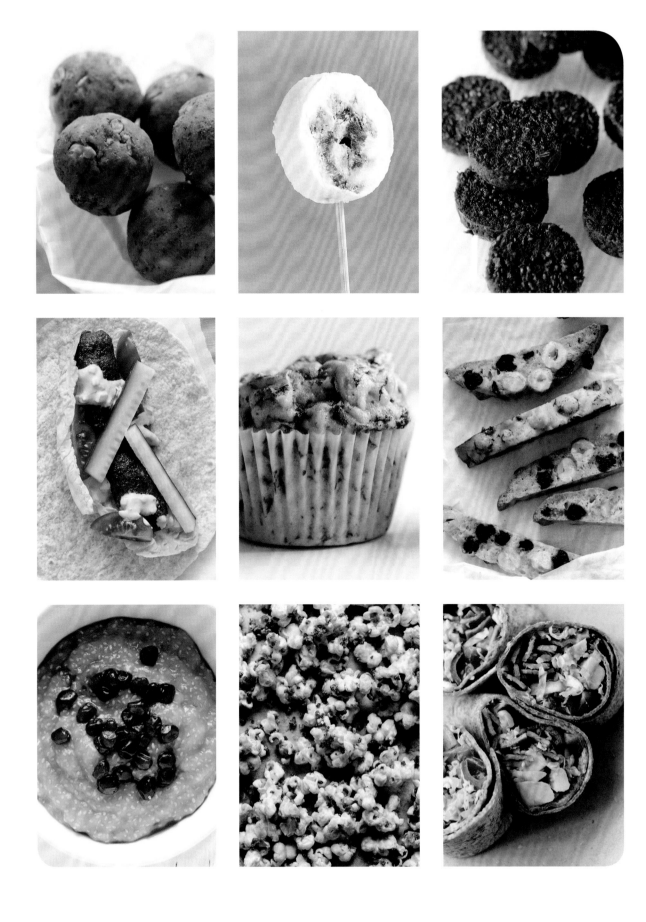

SNACKS

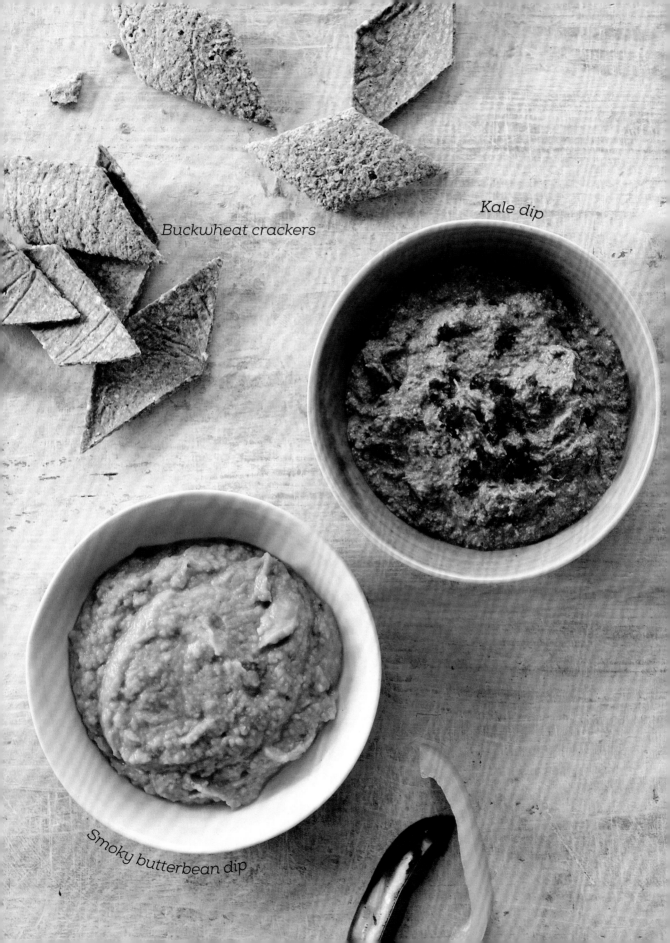

Buckwheat crackers

Kale dip

Smoky butterbean dip

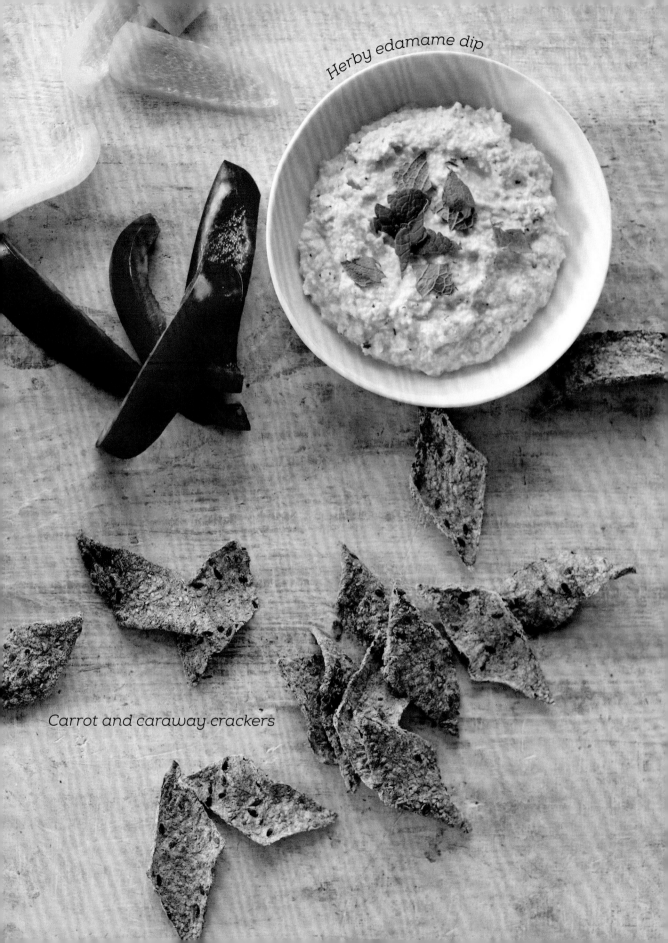

Herby edamame dip

Carrot and caraway crackers

Smoky butter bean dip with carrot and caraway crackers

Ditch the shop-bought tubs and make your own dips. This butter (lima) bean version is rich, creamy and delicious and the crackers make a great alternative to pitta.

Health Butter (lima) beans are a good source of cholesterol-lowering fibre. Plus, they help slow down the rise of blood sugar after a meal.

Top tip If you have any leftover dip, try adding to a salad in place of your usual dressing.

SERVES 4

FOR THE CARROT AND CARAWAY CRACKERS:

250g (9oz) carrot pulp (see pages 230 and 236)

1 tbsp chia seeds

1 tsp caraway seeds

1 tsp fennel seeds

2 tsp ground almonds

a pinch of salt

¼ tsp cracked black pepper

30ml (2 tbsp) water

FOR THE BUTTER BEAN DIP:

400g (14oz) tin butter (lima) beans, drained

1 tsp chipotle paste

50g (scant ¼ cup) quark

100ml (scant ½ cup) skimmed milk

¼ tsp salt, to taste

Preheat the oven to its lowest setting (we used 90°C/194°F), and you'll need a baking tray (cookie sheet).

Mix all the cracker ingredients in a bowl and leave for 30 minutes.

On a work surface, roll the mixture out between 2 sheets of parchment paper until 3–4mm (⅛in) thick. Transfer the sheets, with the mixture between, to the baking tray (cookie sheet) and remove the top sheet of parchment and discard.

Place in a preheated oven for 2 hours. Then, remove from the oven and score the cracker sheet into quarters.

Arrange the crackers on the baking tray again and return to the oven for 3–4 hours until completely dried out. These crackers will keep for 5 days in an airtight container.

Meanwhile, make the dip. Place the butter (lima) beans, chipotle paste and quark into a food processor and blitz until smooth, adding the milk, as required, to achieve the desired consistency. Add salt, to taste, and serve with the crackers.

Kale dip with sugar snap peas

Perfect party food or a guilt-free mid-afternoon snack. The addition of cottage cheese makes this dip creamy and delicious without the extra calories.

Health Kale is a great source of what's known as non-haem iron, providing a perfect iron hit for all vegetarians.

Sport Cottage cheese provides a good hit of casein (slow-release protein), so makes a perfect pre-sleep snack to 'drip-feed' the muscles.

SERVES 2

50g (1¾oz) kale, leaves removed from the stems

150g (⅔ cup) low-fat cottage cheese

1½ tsp roasted garlic paste (see above)

dried chilli (red pepper) flakes, to taste

fresh lemon juice, to taste

150g (5½oz) sugar snap peas, to serve

FOR THE ROASTED GARLIC PASTE:

4 bulbs garlic

Preheat the oven to 180°C/350°F/gas mark 4. First, make the roasted garlic paste. Wrap the bulbs in foil, place on a baking tray (cookie sheet) and roast for 35–40 minutes. To check they're done, open the foil, push the tip of a sharp knife into the side of one bulb, the garlic inside should be golden brown; if not, return to the oven for 10–12 minutes. Remove from the oven and allow to cool a little. Using a pair of scissors, cut the top off each bulb and squeeze the insides out into a ramekin. Use the back of a fork to squash the garlic into a paste and set aside in an airtight container in the fridge. (This keeps for a week in the fridge.)

Steam the kale leaves for 4 minutes. Transfer to a sieve (strainer) and run under cold water for 2–3 minutes until cold. Using the back of a spoon, squeeze out as much water as you can. Put the kale, cottage cheese and roasted garlic paste into a blender and blitz until smooth. Add the chilli and lemon juice, to taste. Serve with sugar snap peas.

Herby edamame dip with buckwheat crackers

Dip into this fresh and fragrant snack as many times as you like guilt free! This edamame dip is flavourful and nutritious and a nice change from regular hummus.

Top tip For a variation, remove the mint leaves and try adding some chilli and a squeeze of lime for tasty Asian flavours.

Sport Edamame is a popular snack among athletes. It's high in protein and one of the few plant foods that contain all the essential amino acids.

SERVES 4

FOR THE BUCKWHEAT CRACKERS (MAKES 8 PORTIONS):

200g (1⅓ cups) whole buckwheat (aka buckwheat groats)

60g (2oz) brown rice protein

2 tsp pink peppercorns

1½ tsp black mustard seeds

1 tbsp extra virgin olive oil

150ml (⅔ cup) water

FOR THE DIP:

250g (9oz) edamame

100g (scant ½ cup) Greek yogurt

2 sprigs mint leaves

5g (⅛oz) coriander (cilantro)

2 tsp extra virgin olive oil

sea salt and freshly ground black pepper, to taste

Preheat the oven to 140°C/275°F/gas mark 1, and line a baking tray (cookie sheet) with baking parchment.

To make the crackers, put all of the dry ingredients into a food processor and blitz until you have a coarse flour consistency. Tip the mixture into a large bowl, add the oil and three-quarters of the water and knead into a dough; you may need to add the rest of the water a little at a time until the dough holds together.

Put a piece of parchment on your work surface and put the dough on top. Using your hands flatten the dough into a roughly rectangular shape. Then, place another sheet of parchment over the top and, using a rolling pin, roll out the dough until it's about 3–4mm (⅛in) thick. Remove the top sheet of parchment, trim the edges to neaten and divide up the dough into 5cm x 3cm (2in x 1¼in) pieces.

Transfer the pieces to the prepared baking tray (cookie sheet) and bake in a preheated oven for 30 minutes. Turn each cracker over and bake for a further 30 minutes or until completely dry. Serve a 30g (1oz) portion of crackers with a quarter the dip.

To make the dip, simply put all the ingredients into a food processor and blitz until smooth; serve immediately.

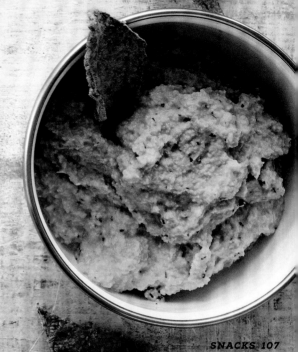

Personalise the snacks with your choice of dipper

○ **Balance** Serve with carrot and caraway crackers.

▽ **Burn** Serve with crudité as dippers.

△ **Build** Serve with buckwheat crackers.

Manchego and chipotle bites

These gluten-free bites are ideal as an appetiser or predinner nibble when you have guests.

Health Sweet potatoes have a lower GI than white potatoes. They're packed with vitamin C and beta-carotene – great for your immunity and vision.

Sport These delicious bites are carb-rich, making them perfect for replenishing glycogen stores after exercise.

MAKES 20/4 PORTIONS

FOR THE BITES:

4 sweet potatoes (a total weight of about 1kg/2lb 4oz)

80g (⅔ cup) Manchego cheese, finely grated

100g (3½oz) sweetcorn

50g (½ cup) buckwheat flour

1 tsp chipotle paste

1 tsp gluten-free baking powder

1 egg

1 tsp salt

FOR THE CORIANDER (CILANTRO) AND LIME YOGURT DIP:

160g (¾ cup) Greek yogurt

finely grated zest of ½ lime

juice of 1 lime

1 tsp agave syrup

10g (¼ cup) coriander (cilantro) leaves, chopped

Preheat the oven to 180°C/350°F/gas mark 4, and line a baking tray (cookie sheet) with baking parchment.

Peel the sweet potatoes and put them through a juicer, remove any larger pieces that have fallen into the pulp. Then, weigh out 180g (6½oz) of the sweet potato pulp into a large bowl.

Add the Manchego cheese followed by the rest of the ingredients and mix thoroughly to form a dough-like consistency.

Roll the dough into 20 walnut-sized balls, arrange on the baking tray (cookie sheet) and bake in a preheated oven for 18–20 minutes.

Meanwhile, make the coriander (cilantro) and lime yogurt dip by mixing all the ingredients together and set aside in a bowl.

Remove the bites from the oven and serve a portion (5 bites) with the zingy dipping sauce on the side.

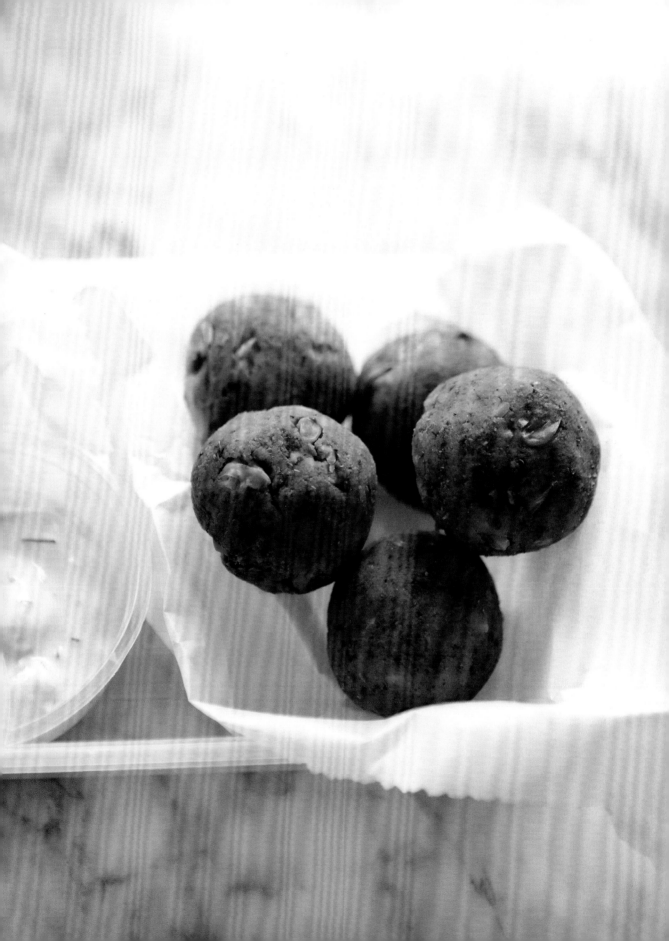

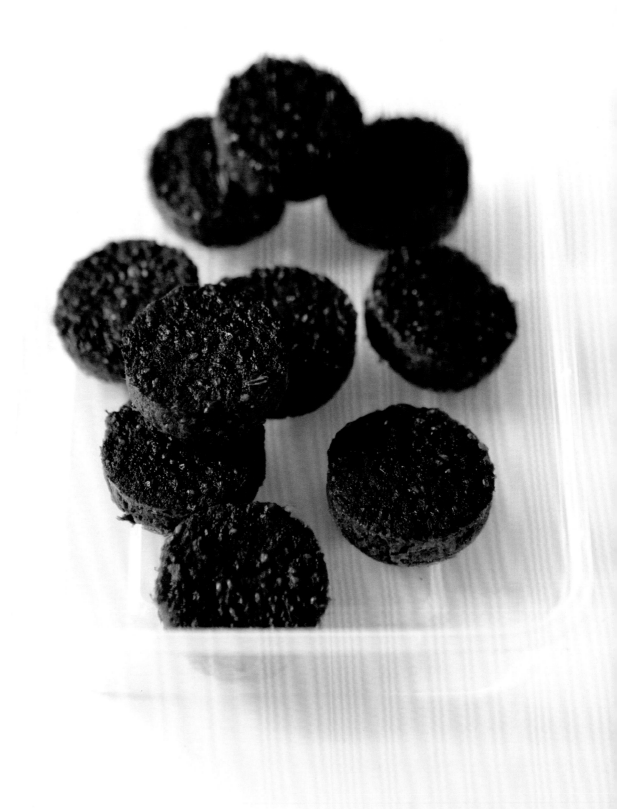

Beetroot turkey bites

These low-carb, low-fat snacks are ideal as an energy boost to fight the afternoon slump.

Health Beetroot is high in vitamins and minerals and packed with age-defying antioxidants.

Sport The turkey and the chia seeds in these little bites mean they are protein packed, which makes them ideal for a pre- or post-training snack.

MAKES 6 PORTIONS

300g (10½oz) raw beetroot

200g (7oz) turkey mince (ground turkey)

30g (scant ¼ cup) chia seeds

2 tsp roasted garlic paste (see page 106)

1 tsp wholegrain mustard

3 eggs

¼ tsp ground white pepper

1cm (½in) cube root ginger, finely chopped

1½ tsp fennel seeds

1 tsp gluten-free baking powder

¾ tsp salt

Peel the beetroots and put them through a juicer, empty the pulp into a bowl and remove any larger pieces that may have fallen in. Weigh out 150g (5½oz) of beetroot pulp; use the juice to make Up beet (see page 229).

Place the pulp with the rest of the ingredients in a bowl and, using a wooden spoon, mix well till bound together. Leave to rest for 1 hour.

Preheat the oven to 170°C/344°F/gas mark 3, and line a baking tray (cookie sheet) with baking parchment or use a silicone baking tray mould (cookie sheet mold) with individual button-shaped recesses.

Transfer the mixture into the moulds or onto the prepared baking tray (cookie sheet) and flatten down with a spatula, as necessary. Bake in a preheated oven for 10–12 minutes.

Remove from the oven, allow to cool for a few minutes and pop out of the moulds or turn the tray over onto a chopping (cutting) board and slice into 2cm- (¾in-) square pieces. One portion is 80g (3¼oz) or about 6 bites.

Lemon cashew bars

A tasty, no-bake bar with minimal preparation that will go down a treat, without being too sweet.

Health Packed full of fibre and monounsaturated fats, these bars are sure to curb any hunger pangs, while satisfying your sweet tooth at the same time.

Sport A great fuelling snack – eat an hour before a training session to give you the quick-release energy to train hard.

MAKES 8

225g (1½ cups) cashews

40g (¼ cup) golden raisins

30g (4½ tsp) agave syrup

finely grated zest and juice of 2 lemons

25g (1oz) puffed quinoa

25g (scant 2 cups) unsweetened puffed rice

Put the cashews and raisins into a food processor and blitz until the mixture starts to stick together. Transfer to a large bowl, stir in the agave syrup and lemon zest and juice with a wooden spoon until well combined, then mix in the puffed quinoa and puffed rice.

Line a baking tray (cookie sheet) with baking parchment and spoon the mixture onto the tray and smooth out, cover the top with another piece of parchment and place a second tray on top. Press the top tray down to compact the mixture and place a weight on top. Chill for 2 hours.

Remove from the fridge, turn out onto a chopping (cutting) board and cut into 8 pieces. One portion is 1 piece.

Gingerbread bites

This easy to make, hand-pressed favourite brings all the flavours of traditional gingerbread without being laden with refined ingredients and heavy fats.

Top tip Enjoy as small bites for snack time or mould into bigger bars for fuelling your workouts.

Health These fibre-packed snacks (thank the dates) will help improve digestion and efficient bowel movement.

MAKES 6 PORTIONS

200g (7oz) pitted dates

50g (⅓ cup) pecans

50g (¼ cup) flaked (slivered) almonds

1 tsp vanilla extract

2 tsp water

½ tsp ground cinnamon

½ tsp ground ginger

50g (½ cup) ground almonds, plus extra for dusting

Preheat the oven to 120°C/250°F/gas mark ½, and you'll need 2 baking trays (cookie sheets), one of which should be lined with baking parchment. Place the dates onto a baking tray (cookie sheet) and bake in the oven for 10–12 minutes until soft. Remove from the oven and set aside. Meanwhile, in a food processor pulse the nuts to a coarse consistency.

Tip the dates into a free-standing food mixer with a beater paddle and work until broken down to a pulp. Add the nuts, vanilla extract, water and spices. Mix until well combined. Slowly add the ground almonds until it comes together to form a firm dough. (If you don't have a food mixer, then mix all of the ingredients in a bowl using your hands (be careful here as the dates will be quite hot, you may need to leave to cool first). Then tip out onto a work surface and knead together until the dates have broken down and you have a dough-like consistency.)

Turn the dough out onto the prepared baking tray (cookie sheet) and press down flat with the back of a spoon. Chill for at least 2 hours. When set, remove from the fridge and turn out onto a chopping (cutting) board. Cut into 36 small cubes, dust with ground almonds and roll the cubes around to coat. Serve 6 cubes or weigh out 60g (2¼oz) to give you a portion. These bites keep for 2 weeks in an airtight container.

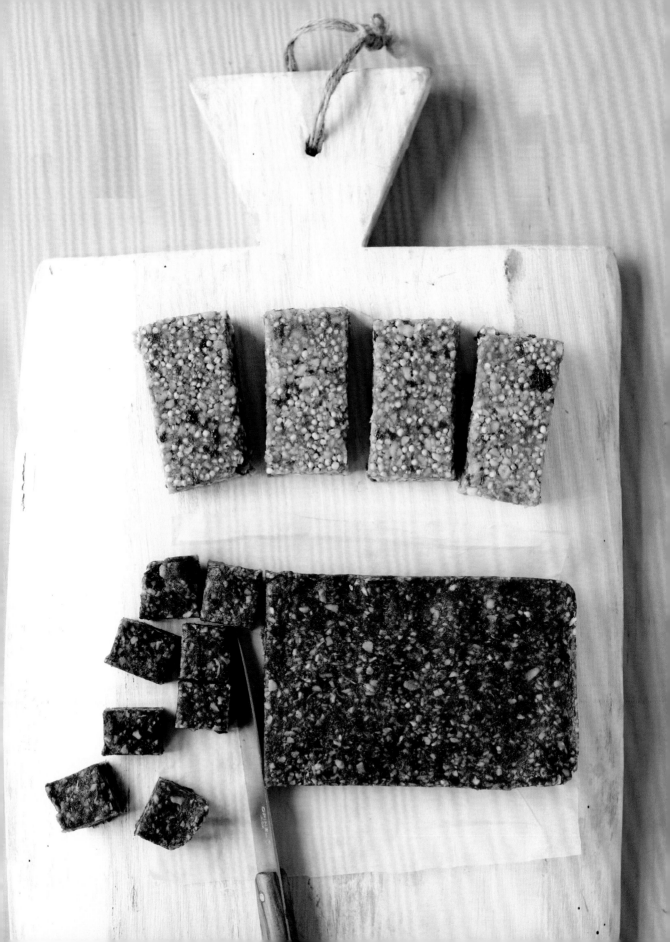

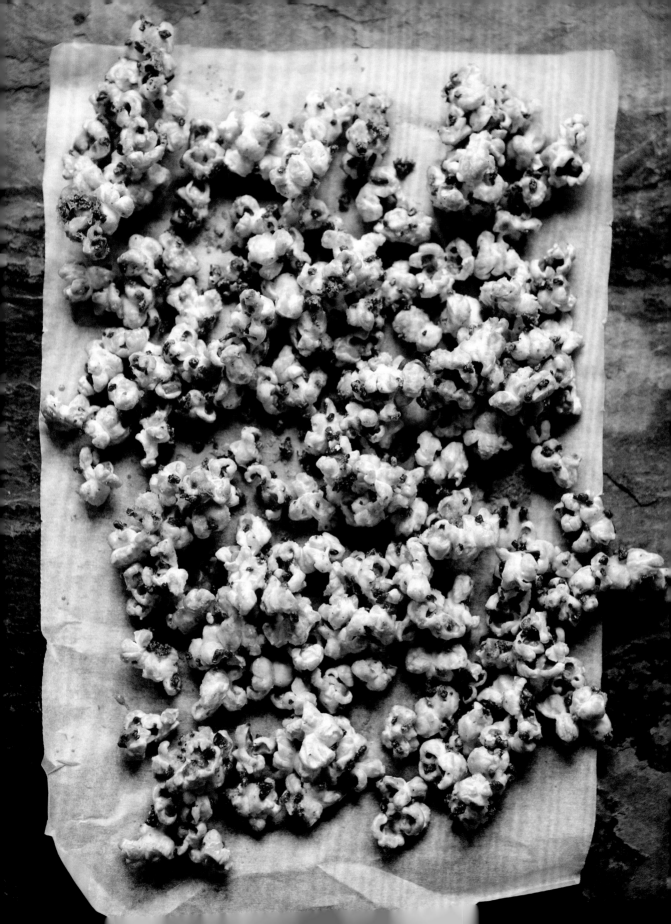

Maple and bacon popcorn

This wonderfully tasty popcorn is healthy and nutritious, despite appearances. The smoky bacon and maple syrup make this a sweet and salty addictive bowl of popcorn you will not want to share!

Health Coconut oil is the most nutrient-dense part of a coconut. It's a wonderful way of increasing the healthy fats in your diet.

Sport The zinc found in maple syrup helps maintain strong immunity whatever your training demands.

SERVES 4

4 rashers (slices) smoked back (Canadian) bacon

100g (⅓ cup) maple syrup

1 tsp coconut oil

50g (¼ cup) popcorn kernels

Preheat the oven to 160°C/325°F/gas mark 2½.

Trim all the fat from the bacon and finely mince (grind) it. Put it on a non-stick baking tray (cookie sheet) and bake in a preheated oven for 15–20 minutes. Give it a stir around every 5 minutes until crispy and brown. When done, remove from the oven and turn the heat down to 120°C/250°F/gas mark ½. Heat the maple syrup in a pan over a medium heat and reduce it by half.

Meanwhile, place the oil and popcorn kernels in a large pan with a lid. Put the lid on and shake until the corn is coated with the oil. Put the pan on a low to medium heat and wait a few minutes for the corn to start popping. When the popping has slowed to less than 1 pop per 5 seconds, remove from the heat (at this point you can pick out any unpopped kernels if you wish) and pour in the reduced syrup and mix in the crispy bacon. Mix well and transfer to a baking tray (cookie sheet). Bake in a preheated oven for a further 15–20 minutes. Divide into quarters to serve and hand out to friends, or keep in an airtight container for 5 days.

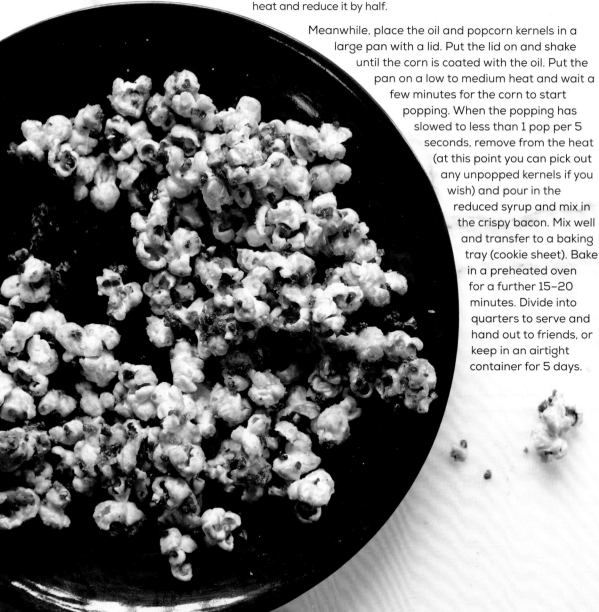

Parmesan and sunblush tomato biscuits

You may not have thought of combining the flavours found in this snack but, believe us, it works fabulously well. Keep these savoury snacks in an airtight container or pop a batch in the freezer for later.

Health This combination of ingredients covers many nutritional bases including sources of calcium, monounsaturated fats and vitamin C.

Top tip These biscuits (cookies) freeze well so if you have made too many don't worry! Simply wrap in clingfilm (plastic wrap) and place in the freezer.

MAKES 10

1 egg

100g (7 tbsp) spreadable light butter

½ tsp baking powder

175g (1¼ cups) plain all-purpose) flour

50g (½ cup) walnuts, crushed

50g (1¾oz) sunblush tomatoes, chopped

20g (¼ cup) sunflower seeds

30g (1oz) spinach, chopped

½ tsp thyme, leaves picked and chopped

50g (½ cup) Parmesan cheese, finely grated

In a free-standing food mixer with a beater paddle, or a large bowl and wooden spoon, beat the egg into the light butter. Add the rest of the ingredients and mix well.

Lay out a double layer of clingfilm (plastic wrap) (about 60cm/23in wide) on a work surface. Spoon the mixture onto the edge closest to you in a rough sausage shape. Now, roll it up and then tie the ends, twisting to tighten. Allow to rest in the fridge for at least 1 hour.

Meanwhile, preheat the oven to 170°C/344°F/gas mark 3, and line a baking tray (cookie sheet) with baking parchment.

Remove the 'dough log' from the fridge and cut it into 10 slices, discarding a little at the ends. Lay the slices on the prepared tray and bake in the oven for 15–20 minutes. When done, remove from the oven and cool on a wire rack. One biscuit (cookie) equals 1 snack portion.

Reheating frozen biscuits (cookies): when you are ready to reheat, pop the biscuits on a baking tray (cookie sheet) and place in a preheated oven (160°C/325°F/gas mark 2½) for 8–10 minutes to crisp up.

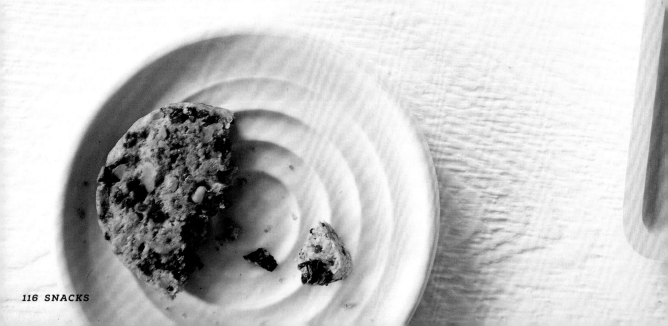

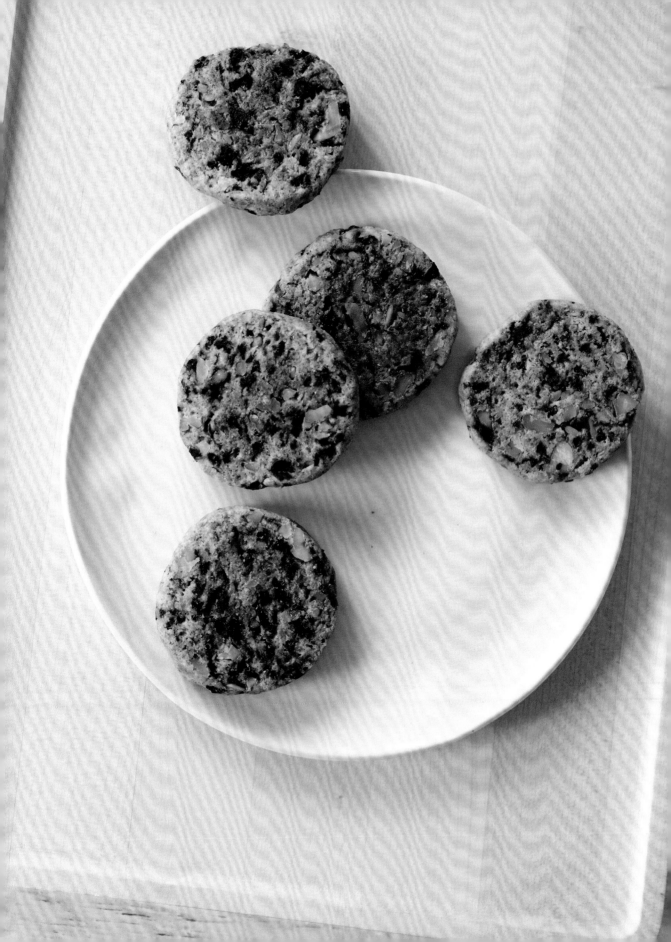

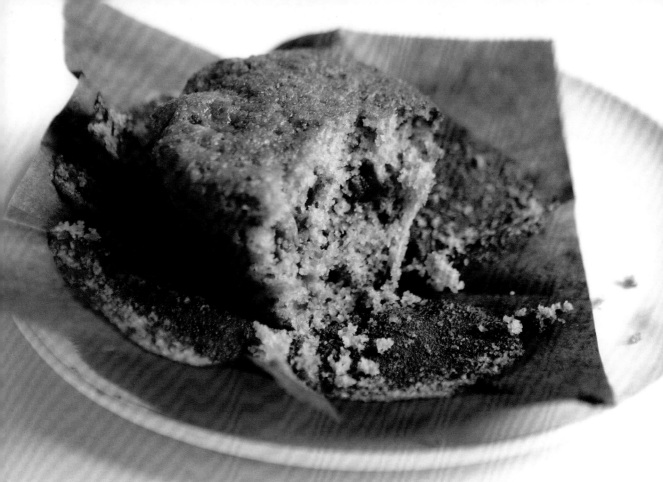

Violet and raspberry muffins

Muffins don't have to be heavy and sugary, made well they can be tasty, light and – best of all – better for you. These violet and raspberry muffins are truly delicious.

Health Not only are these muffins protein rich, but they're also packed with antioxidant-rich fruit.

Top tip Experiment with flavours – use vanilla extract and cranberries for a seasonal twist.

MAKES 6

60ml (¼ cup) skimmed milk
4 drops violet essence (extract)
75g (½ cup) gluten-free flour
50g (1¾oz) unflavoured whey protein
1 tsp gluten-free baking powder
55g (4 tbsp) spreadable light butter
115g (½ cup + 2 tbsp) coconut palm sugar
1 egg
150g (1¼ cups) raspberries, crushed

Preheat the oven to 180°C/350°F/gas mark 4, and line a 6- or 12-hole muffin tin with 6 paper cases.

Using a beaker and hand-held blender, blend together the milk and the violet essence (extract).

In a bowl, mix the flour and protein and baking powders together.

Then, in a large bowl using an electric whisk, cream the light butter and coconut palm sugar together until light and fluffy, then beat in the egg.

Mix half of the dry mixture into the butter–egg mix followed by half of the milk, then repeat with the remaining halves until thoroughly combined. Lastly, using a spatula fold in the crushed raspberries.

Bake in a preheated oven for 18–20 minutes. The muffins are ready when a skewer inserted into the centre of one comes out clean.

Remove from the oven, allow to cool in the tin for 10 minutes then transfer to a wire rack. These will keep in an airtight container for 3 days.

Pesto and polenta protein muffins

Who says muffins have to be sweet? This scrumptious mix of pesto and polenta may just change your opinion of savoury muffins. Baked until golden brown, these muffins are a real delight!

Top tip Enjoy these muffins warm. If you are not planning to eat them straightaway, they keep really well in an airtight container in the fridge.

Sport These muffins are perfect for a post-training snack. The combo of whey protein and polenta will help to replenish carb stores and rebuild muscle.

MAKES 6

- 100g (3½oz) baby spinach leaves
- 30g (¾ cup) basil
- 1 egg
- 25g (¼ cup) Parmesan cheese, grated
- 55ml (¼ cup) extra virgin olive oil
- 2 cloves garlic
- 45g (⅓ cup) pine nuts
- 45g (1½oz) unflavoured whey protein
- 65g (½ cup) polenta (cornmeal)
- ¼ tsp xanthan gum
- 1½ tsp gluten-free baking powder
- 5g (⅛oz) organic vegetable bouillon (½ cube or 1½ tsp powder)
- ½ tsp salt
- ¼ tsp ground white pepper
- 2 egg whites

Preheat the oven to 180°C/350°F/gas mark 4, and line a 6- or 12-hole muffin tin with 6 paper cases.

Boil some water in a large pan . Drop the spinach and basil into the water for 30 seconds, then drain and chill in a bowl of iced water. Drain into a sieve (strainer) and squeeze with the back of a large spoon. Finely chop both, then add along with the rest of the ingredients, except for the egg whites, to a large bowl and, using a spatula, mix together.

In another large bowl using an electric whisk, whisk the egg whites to form soft peaks. Next, gently fold the egg whites into the spinach mixture and divide between the lined muffin cases.

Bake in a preheated oven for 18–20 minutes. The muffins are ready when a skewer inserted into the centre of one comes out clean.

Remove from the oven, allow to cool in the tin for 10 minutes then transfer to a wire rack. Store any muffins not scoffed while warm in an airtight container and store in the fridge until you're ready to eat.

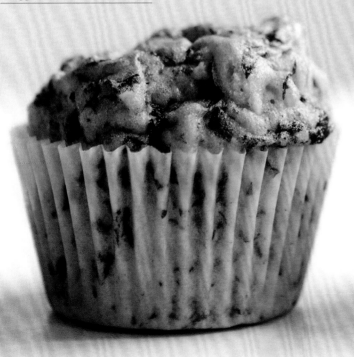
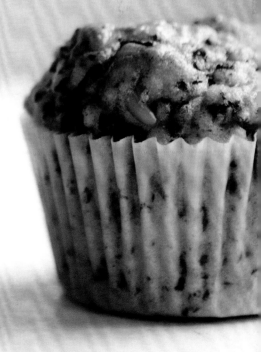

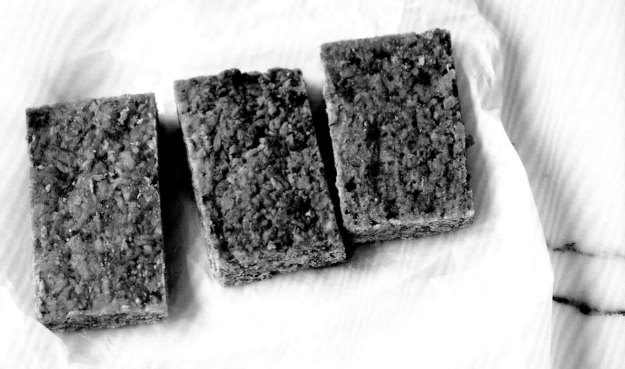

Orange and ginger flapjacks

The flapjack as you know it but with a healthy twist and a zesty kick. Perfect for big-batch making and sharing with your friends and family.

Health This sweet treat comes with an immunity boost! The antibacterial properties of ginger and honey make this a good snack for avoiding colds.

Sport Great to keep handy when out and about, at the training ground or in your gym for when you need an energy boost or after a particularly hard session.

MAKES 15

375g (1 cup) honey

375g (1⅔ cups) spreadable light butter

600g (10½ cups) flaked oats

30g (1oz) unflavoured whey protein

finely grated zest of 1 orange

50g (1¾oz) stem (preserved) ginger, finely chopped

Preheat the oven to 160°C/325°F/gas mark 2½, and line a baking tray (cookie sheet) with baking parchment.

Melt the honey and light butter in a large pan on a low heat. Remove from the heat, add the oats, protein, orange zest and stem (preserved) ginger, and mix well with a wooden spoon.

Turn the mixture out onto the prepared baking tray (cookie sheet) and bake in a preheated oven for 20–25 minutes until golden. Remove from the oven and allow to cool.

Turn the flapjack out onto a chopping (cutting) board and divide into 15 pieces. One piece equals a portion for a snack. This flapjack keeps for 7 days in an airtight container.

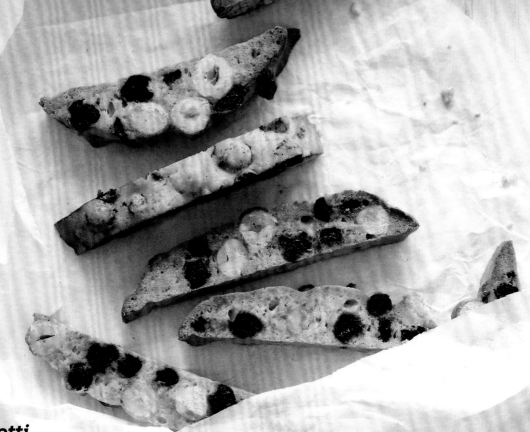

Biscotti

This crunchy, crumbly goodness is perfect served alongside a steaming hot cup of coffee! Sure to give you a sweet fix without piling on the pounds.

Top tip Try using Montmorency cherries instead of the blueberries – they taste delicious and can help ease muscle pain following exercise.

Sport This protein-filled snack is low in fat and sugar – so is great for after a workout.

SERVES 8

60g (scant ½ cup) wholemeal (wholewheat) flour

60g (2¼oz) unflavoured whey protein

90g (¼ cup) clear honey

finely grated zest of ½ lemon

½ tsp vanilla extract

¾ tsp gluten-free baking powder

2 eggs

130g (generous ¾ cup) dried blueberries

70g (½ cup) hazelnuts

Preheat the oven to 160°C/325°F/gas mark 2½, and line 2 baking trays (cookie sheets) with baking parchment.

Mix the flour, protein, honey, lemon zest, vanilla extract and baking powder together in a large bowl.

Whisk the eggs a little, then mix into the ingredients in the bowl, adding a little at a time until a dough is formed. Lastly, add the blueberries and hazelnuts and mix in well.

Split the dough in half and roll each into a rough sausage shape about 15cm (6in) long. Place each onto a prepared baking tray (cookie sheet) and cook in a preheated oven for 18-20 minutes until firm.

Remove from the oven and allow to cool for a few minutes. Meanwhile, turn the oven down to its lowest setting.

Using a large serrated knife, slice the biscuit (cookie) 'sausages' into 1cm- (½in-) thick slices and arrange the slices on the trays. Return to the oven for a further 70–80 minutes or until completely dried out. These biscotti keep for 3–5 days in an airtight container.

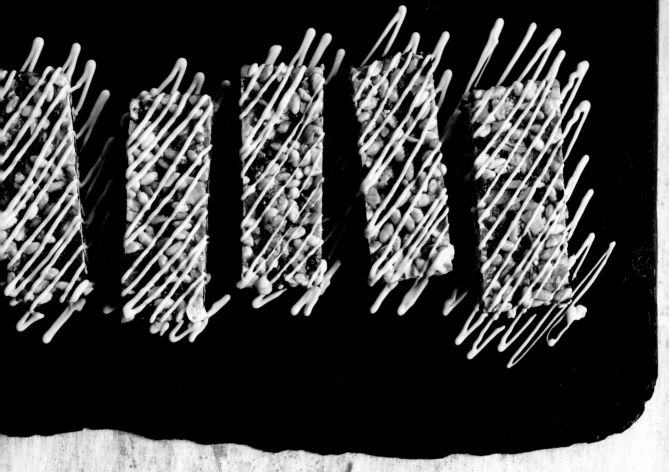

Apricot and chocolate puffed rice bars

This delicious, sticky, sweet bar will help to curb those sugar cravings. Plus, the puffed rice will help to keep you satisfied inbetween meals.

Health The beta-carotene content of dried apricots makes them especially rich in vitamin A, which is essential for cell regrowth.

Sport Enjoy this yummy bar as a superb post-training pick-me-up.

MAKES 6

160g (½ cup) honey

20g desiccated coconut

25g (¼ cup) flaked (slivered) almonds

75g (½ cup) dried apricots

15g cocoa nibs

30g (1oz) unsweetened puffed rice

½ tsp vanilla extract

50g (1¾oz) white chocolate

Line a 450g (1lb) loaf tin with baking parchment.

In a small pan over a medium heat reduce the honey by half.

Put the rest of the ingredients, apart from the white chocolate, into a large bowl and pour over the hot honey. Mix well using a wooden spoon until everything is well coated.

Spoon the mixture into the prepared tin and place another piece of baking parchment on top. Use your hands to firmly push the mixture into all the corners and until the surface is even. Chill in the fridge for 2 hours.

Remove from the tin, place on a chopping (cutting) board, strip off the parchment and slice into 6 portions.

Finally, melt the chocolate in the microwave on low power for 15 seconds at a time (about 1 minute in total). Pour the melted chocolate into a piping (pastry) bag and, using a small nozzle (tip), drizzle equally over the pieces.

The ultimate power bar

This healthy energy bar will be your saving grace when you're in need of a 3.30pm pick-me up or mid-morning energy boost. It's the ultimate combination of good fats, carbs and protein to fuel your daily duties.

Health Puffed quinoa is a great addition to add to raw energy bars. It is high in complete protein and has twice as much fibre as most other grains.

Top tip Cut into small-cube-sized pieces and enjoy a couple for a mini-energy-lift while you're on the go.

MAKES 8

- 40g (3 tbsp) coconut oil
- 40g (1½oz) puffed quinoa
- 40g (¼ cup) whole buckwheat (aka buckwheat groats)
- 40g (⅓ cup) cocoa nibs
- 40g (⅓ cup) pumpkin seeds
- 40g (¼ cup) dried blueberries
- 40g (⅓ cup) dried cranberries
- ½ tsp vanilla extract
- 75g (2½oz) unflavoured whey protein
- 2 tsp cocoa powder
- 2 tbsp honey
- 4 tsp xylitol
- 1 egg, lightly beaten
- 30ml (2 tbsp) water

Preheat the oven to 160°C/325°F/gas mark 2½, and line an 18cm (7in) square loose-bottomed cake tin with baking parchment.

In a small pan melt the coconut oil.

Put the rest of the ingredients in a large bowl and, using a wooden spoon, mix thoroughly. Mix in the oil until well combined.

Transfer the mixture to the prepared cake tin and smooth down using the back of the spoon. Bake in a preheated oven for 15 minutes until firm. Then, remove from the oven, allow to cool in the tin briefly and then transfer to a wire rack. Once cooled, turn out onto a chopping (cutting) board and cut into 8 pieces. Serve 1 piece as 1 portion.

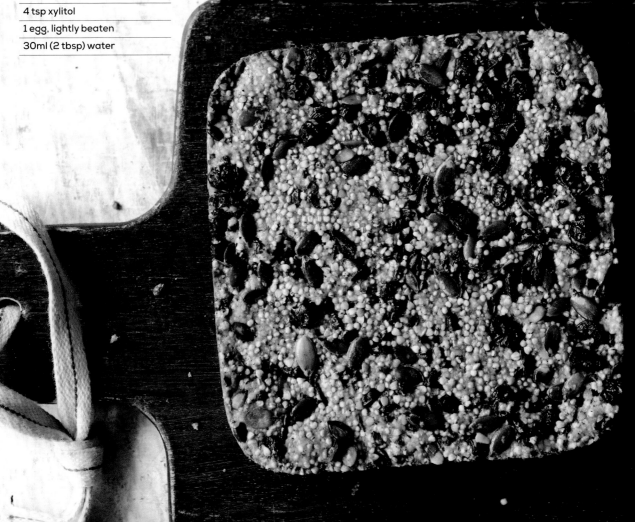

Millionaire's shortbread

A healthy take on this classic British treat – bittersweet chocolate and crumbly shortbread, sandwiched together with a sticky, sweet cheat of date caramel.

Health Thanks to the quark, it is far lower in fat than the usual treat. Quark has a high source of casein, making it a great way to feed muscles, too.

Top tip Do you like thicker shortbread and caramel layers? Make this treat in a 15cm (6in) square tin and bake the shortbread for 5–7 minutes longer.

MAKES 12

110g (¾ cup) wholemeal (wholewheat) flour

60g (½ cup) cornflour (cornstarch)

60g (⅓ cup) golden caster (superfine) sugar

110g (½ cup) unsalted butter, diced

240g (8½oz) pitted dates

150g (⅔ cup) quark

100g (3½oz) dark chocolate (minimum 70% cocoa solids)

Preheat the oven to 170°C/344°F/gas mark 3, and grease and line an 18cm (7in) square loose-bottomed cake tin (line just the bottom).

Put the flours and sugar into the bowl of a food processor. Turn on to the slowest speed and slowly add the butter until you achieve a breadcrumb-like texture. Tip out onto a work surface and gently knead until it comes together; be careful not to overwork.

Transfer the dough into the prepared tin and press down until evenly distributed around the tin. Allow to rest for 20 minutes.

Bake in a preheated oven for 20 minutes until almost firm in the middle. Remove from the oven and allow to cool for at least 10 minutes.

Meanwhile, warm the dates on a baking tray (cookie sheet) in the oven for 5–6 minutes then transfer to a food processor. Blitz for 1 minute then add the quark and blitz again until quite smooth.

Spoon the date mixture onto the shortbread base, then place a piece of baking parchment on top and press down until evenly spread. Peel off and discard the parchment.

Melt the chocolate in a heatproof bowl over a pan of simmering water. Once melted, pour the chocolate on top of the date mixture and use a spatula to spread out to cover the surface. Chill for 1 hour.

When you're ready to serve, remove from the tin, transfer to a chopping (cutting) board and cut into 12 pieces.

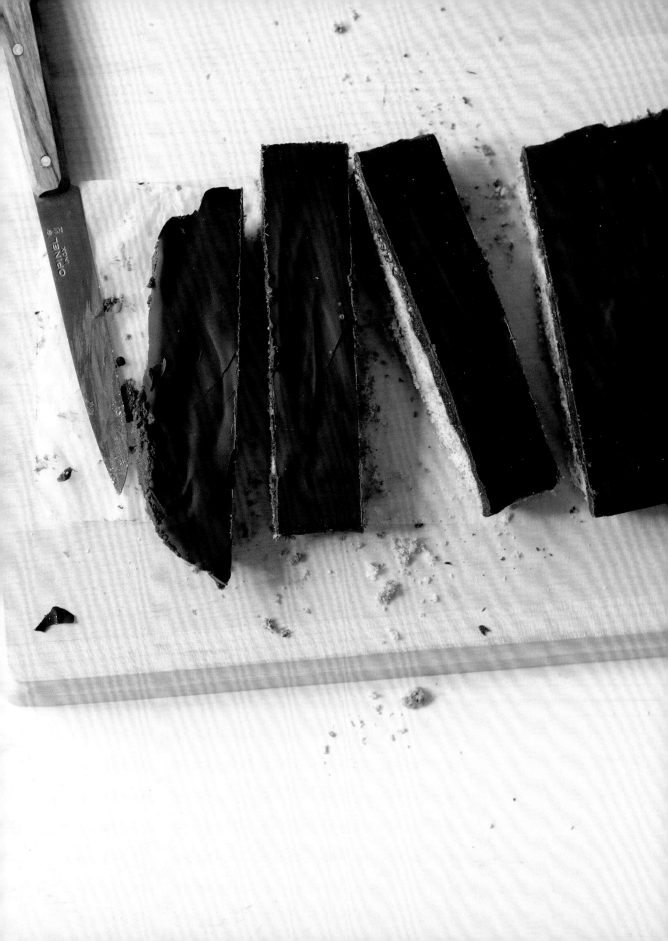

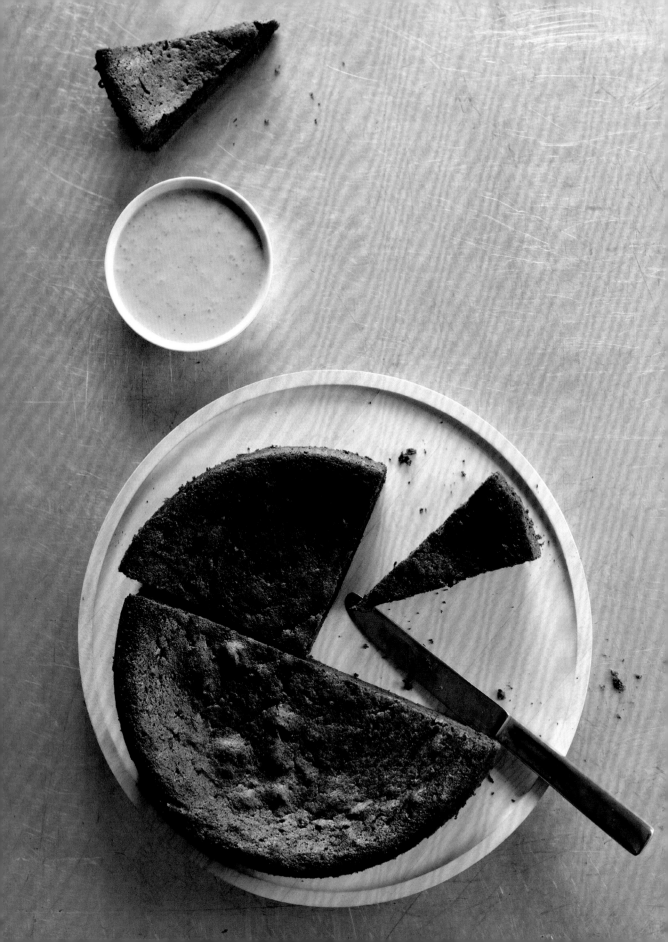

Flourless chocolate cake with pistachio butter

This is a great recipe for those who suffer from intolerance to wheat or gluten. It's super-moist and chocolatey – a real treat without being too naughty.

Top tip If you don't like the sound of the pistachio butter, why not try using the Strawberry cream cheese from page 83 instead.

Sport With the extra hit of hemp powder and the eggs (which contain all the essential amino acids), this snack is a great go-to for muscle growth and repair.

SERVES 8

FOR THE PISTACHIO BUTTER:

70g (½ cup) pistachio nut kernels

50g (2 tbsp) almond butter

1½ tsp honey

FOR THE CAKE:

80g (3¼oz) dark chocolate (minimum 70% cocoa solids)

75g (5½ tbsp) coconut oil

4 eggs, separated

40g (scant ¼ cup) xylitol

25g (1oz) hemp powder

1 tsp bicarbonate of soda (baking soda)

1 tsp cocoa powder

In a blender, blitz the pistachio nuts with the almond butter and honey till smooth. Keep in an airtight container. Serve a 20g (¾oz) portion of this butter per portion of cake.

Preheat the oven to 170°C/344°F/gas mark 3, and grease a 20cm (8in) round springform cake tin.

Melt the chocolate and coconut oil together in a small heatproof bowl over a pan of simmering water.

In a large bowl using an electric whisk or free-standing food mixer, whisk the egg yolks and xylitol together until light and fluffy. When you turn the mixer off and pull it out of the bowl, the mixture that drips off should hold for a few seconds before sinking back into the bowl.

Using a spatula, gently fold the melted chocolate mixture into the egg mix. Then, fold in the rest of the dry ingredients until well combined.

In another bowl, whisk the egg whites to form soft peaks and gently fold into the mixture you have already. Pour this cake mixture into the prepared tin and bake in a preheated oven for 25 minutes.

Remove from the oven, allow to cool in the tin briefly before transferring to a wire rack. Cut into 8 portions when cooled.

Beetroot brownies

Chocolate has great health benefits and can help keep hunger pangs at bay. Marry it up with some sweet beetroot and you've got a super-tasty snack or dessert, to glam up with some zesty yogurt and oaty sprinkles.

Health Chocolate with a high percentage of cocoa solids (80% and over) can help control blood sugar levels and is a great mood lifter, too.

Sport The high levels of protein and moderate carbohydrate make this an ideal post-training recovery snack.

MAKES 10

125g (4½oz) cooked beetroot (we use vacuum-packed in natural juices)

125g (9 tbsp) spreadable light butter

125g (4½oz) dark chocolate (minimum 70% cocoa solids)

2 large eggs

65g (¼ cup + 2 tbsp) soft brown sugar

60g (scant ⅓ cup) xylitol

75g (½ cup) wholemeal self-raising (wholewheat self-rising) flour

FOR THE OATY SPRINKLES:

100g (generous 1 cup) rolled oats

10g (1½ tsp) agave syrup

½ tsp ground cinnamon

FOR THE ORANGE YOGURT (MAKES ENOUGH FOR 10 PORTIONS):

550g (scant 2½ cups) Greek yogurt

12g (⅓oz) orange zest

20ml (4 tsp) orange juice

75g (⅓ cup) agave syrup

50g (1¾oz) unflavoured whey protein

Preheat the oven to 180°C/350°F/gas mark 4, and line a 30cm x 15cm (12in x 6in) (or similar dimensions) baking tray (cookie sheet).

Drain any liquid from the beetroots and, using the coarse side of a cheese grater, grate them into a bowl.

Next, in a heatproof bowl over a pan of simmering water melt the light butter and chocolate together, and set aside.

Using an electric mixer, beat the eggs, sugar and xylitol together until they are light and fluffy. You'll know when it's the right consistency when you turn the mixer off and pull it out of the bowl, the mix that drips off should hold for a few seconds before sinking back into the bowl.

Gently fold the chocolate–butter mixture into the eggs and sugar using a spatula. Then, fold in the flour followed by the beetroot.

Pour the mixture into the prepared baking tray (cookie sheet), it should settle to be about 1–1.5cm (½–⅝in) thick. Bake in the oven for 20–25 minutes. The brownies are done when a skewer inserted into the centre of the bake comes out with only a few crumbs on it. Err on the side of caution as these brownies come out better underdone than overdone.

Remove from the oven and allow to cool in the tin before turning out onto a chopping (cutting) board and cutting into 10 pieces.

For the oaty sprinkles, mix everything together and bake on a baking tray in a preheated oven for 5 minutes until golden brown. Remove from the oven, allow to cool and set aside.

In a bowl, mix all the orange yogurt ingredients together with a spoon until an even consistency is achieved. Serve 1 tablespoon of the orange yogurt and 15g (½oz) of the oaty sprinkles with each portion of brownie.

Burn Follow the recipe above but substitute ground almonds (a low-carb flour) for the self-raising (self-rising) flour when making the brownies.

Balance Omit the oaty sprinkles.

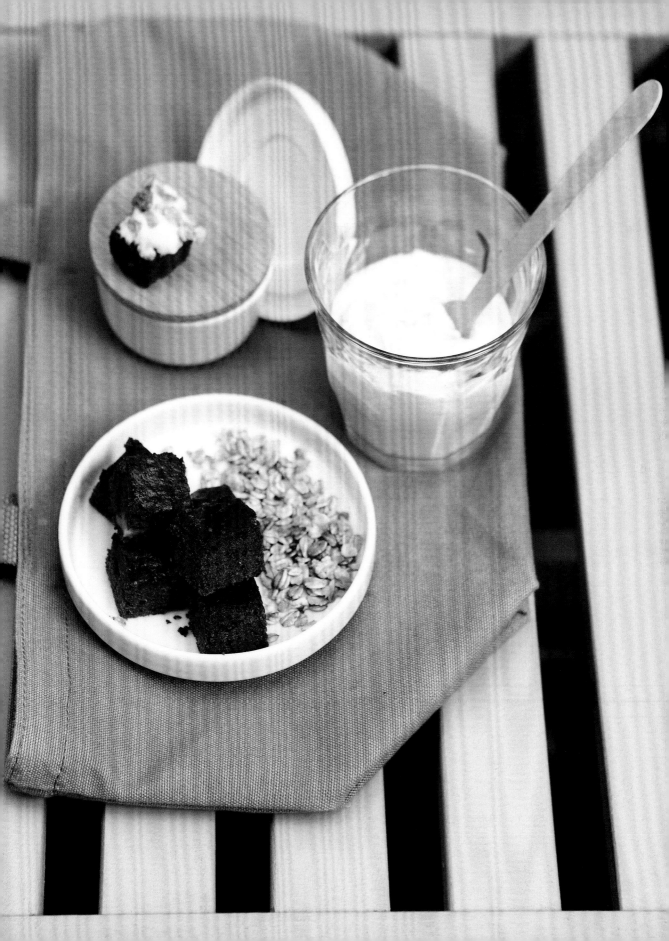

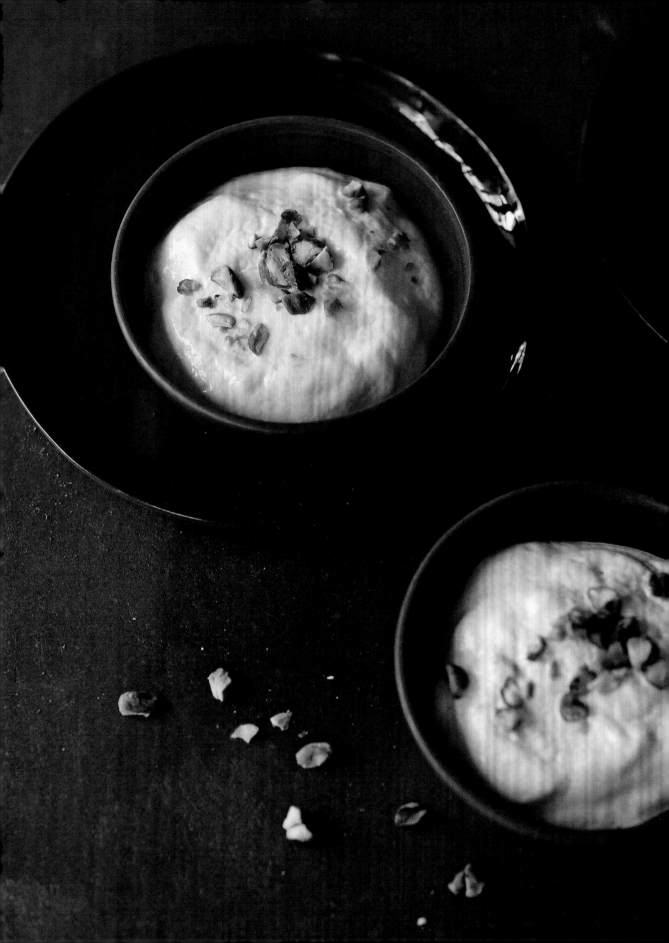

Saffron and honey mousse with crushed pistachios

This quick and easy snack also doubles up as a dinner party dessert (bonus!). And while you're enjoying its Middle Eastern flavours, it'll be doing your middle favours – enjoy this snack on the Burn diet code.

Health Greek yogurt does much more than curb your hunger, it's also a great source of calcium, which is key to strong bones and healthy teeth.

Sport This snack contains a good hit of protein, from the Greek yogurt and pistachios, making this a soporific pre-bedtime snack.

SERVES 2

1 small egg white

1 tsp water

about 15 strands saffron

150g (⅔ cup) Greek yogurt

25g (2 tbsp) honey

25g (scant ¼ cup) pistachio kernels, crushed

In a bowl, mix the egg white together with the water and the saffron. Leave to infuse for 30 minutes.

Meanwhile, mix the yogurt and honey together in a separate bowl.

Strain the saffron and egg white mixture through a fine sieve (strainer) into a bowl. Whisk the egg white with a balloon whisk or electric whisk until it forms soft peaks. Then use a wooden spoon to gently fold the egg white into the yogurt and honey, being very careful not to overmix as you want the mousse to be as light as possible.

To serve, divide the mousse between 2 bowls or glasses and sprinkle over some crushed pistachios.

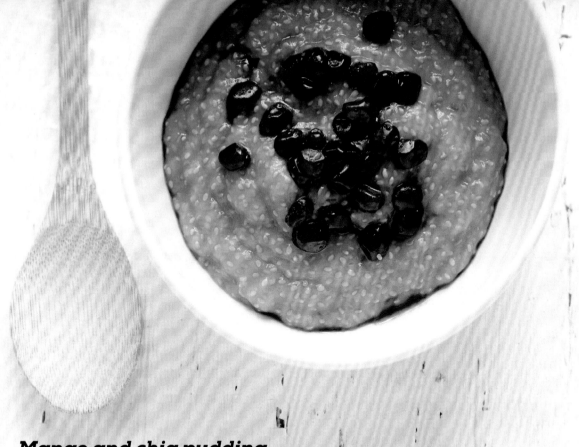

Mango and chia pudding

Super-charge your morning, afternoon or pre-workout energy levels with this exotic treat that's quick to make. It tastes like a tropical paradise and the texture is oh-so delicate. We bet you won't be able to get enough.

Top tip If you'd rather a creamy taste, replace the orange juice with coconut milk and a splash of water for a delicious alternative.

Health Chia seeds are particularly high in omega-3 fatty acids, which makes them highly nutritious and helps to lower blood pressure.

SERVES 2

1 mango
100ml (scant ½ cup) freshly squeezed orange juice
40g (¼ cup) chia seeds
60g (2¼oz) pomegranate seeds

Peel and stone the mango. Then, using a beaker and hand-held blender, blitz the mango into a smooth purée.

Stir in the orange juice and chia seeds and leave in the fridge for 1 hour.

Divide between 2 bowls or glasses and top with pomegranate seeds.

Raspberry and coconut cheesecake lollipops

Don't save these low-fat cheesecake lollipops for the kids, they're great for anyone who is young at heart.

Health This very-low-fat frozen treat also gives you a quick protein fix. So, enjoy knowing it's doing your body good as well.

Top tip As well as making lollies, you can enjoy this snack as an alternative to ice cream. Place the square in the freezer until fully frozen and use one scoop per portion.

SERVES 8

60g (¼ cup) low-fat cream cheese

50g (scant ¼ cup) quark

25g (3½ tsp) agave syrup

40ml (1½ tbsp) low-fat coconut milk

½ tsp xanthan gum

50g (scant ½ cup) raspberries

2 ginger snap biscuits (cookies)

8 bamboo skewers (you just use the pointy end of each)

Using a beaker and a hand-held blender blitz the cream cheese, quark, agave syrup, coconut milk and xanthan gum together until smooth and thoroughly mixed.

In a small bowl or ramekin, crush the raspberries a little with the back of a fork. Break the biscuits (cookies) into small pieces.

Tear off 2 sheets of clingfilm (plastic wrap), about 40cm (16in) square, and lay out on a tray on your work surface.

Pour the cheesecake mixture on top of this and spread out into a square, roughly 15cm (6in). Sprinkle the raspberries and biscuit (cookie) pieces over evenly and pop the tray and mix in the freezer for 20 minutes.

Remove from the freezer, roll the wrapped parcel up into a sausage shape and tie at both ends. Then return to the freezer until thoroughly frozen. Meanwhile, using scissors, cut the skewers down to half the size.

Take the frozen mixture out of the freezer and place on a chopping (cutting) board. Slice into 8 portions using a serrated knife and remove the clingfilm (plastic wrap) from each slice (or cut the lollies out with a small biscuit/cookie cutter). Push the pointy end of each skewer into the side edge of each lolly and serve (trim the skewer as necessary). If you're not serving all the lollies, then refreeze in an airtight container.

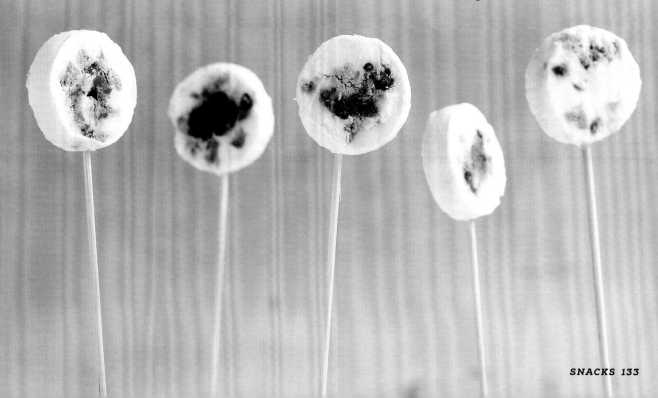

Lamb koftas with beetroot tzatziki

This snack is always a winner with my friends, as it's full of flavour and has a twist on the run-of-the-mill tzatziki. Make a batch and share them out after a training session or a match.

Health Sumac has been found to reduce blood glucose levels, which will help prevent long-term health conditions such as diabetes and obesity.

Top tip Why not make the mince mixture the night before – the spices get to mingle. Just cover the bowl with clingfilm (plastic wrap) and pop it in the fridge.

MAKES 6

FOR THE KOFTAS:

300g (10½oz) lamb mince (ground lamb)

finely grated zest of ½ lemon

½ tsp cumin

½ tsp paprika

½ tsp sumac

¼ tsp dried chilli (red pepper) flakes

1 clove garlic, finely chopped

½ tsp ground allspice

¾ tsp sea salt

¼ tsp ground black pepper

6 wooden skewers

FOR THE BEETROOT TZATZIKI:

¼ cucumber, deseeded

120g (½ cup) low-fat Greek yogurt

½ clove garlic, very finely chopped

6 mint leaves, chopped

a pinch of salt, to taste

10g (⅓oz) beetroot, juiced, or 8ml beetroot juice

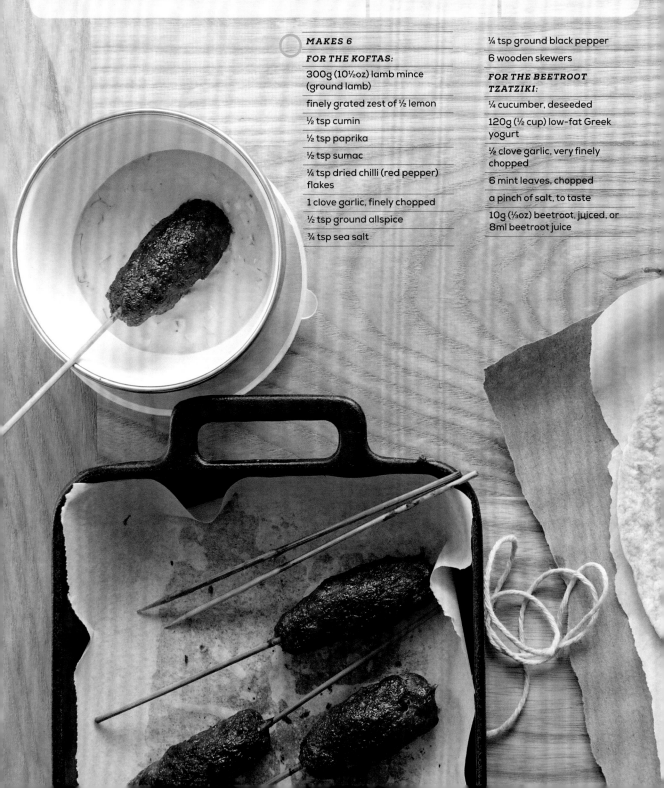

First, make the beetroot tzatziki. Dice the cucumber into small cubes (1cm/½in), and in a bowl mix with the rest of the ingredients. Place in the fridge and leave for 30 minutes before serving.

Preheat the oven to 180°C/350°F/gas mark 4, and line a baking tray (cookie sheet) with baking parchment.

Put all of the koftas ingredients into a bowl and mix together using a wooden spoon until all are well combined.

Divide the mixture into 6 and roll each portion into a sausage shape. Then, push a skewer into the end of each kofta and bake in a preheated oven for 10–12 minutes.

Serve 3 koftas per portion with the tzatziki.

Burn Serve 2 koftas per portion.

Build Serve 3 koftas per portion, plus add a tortilla wrap filled with salad.

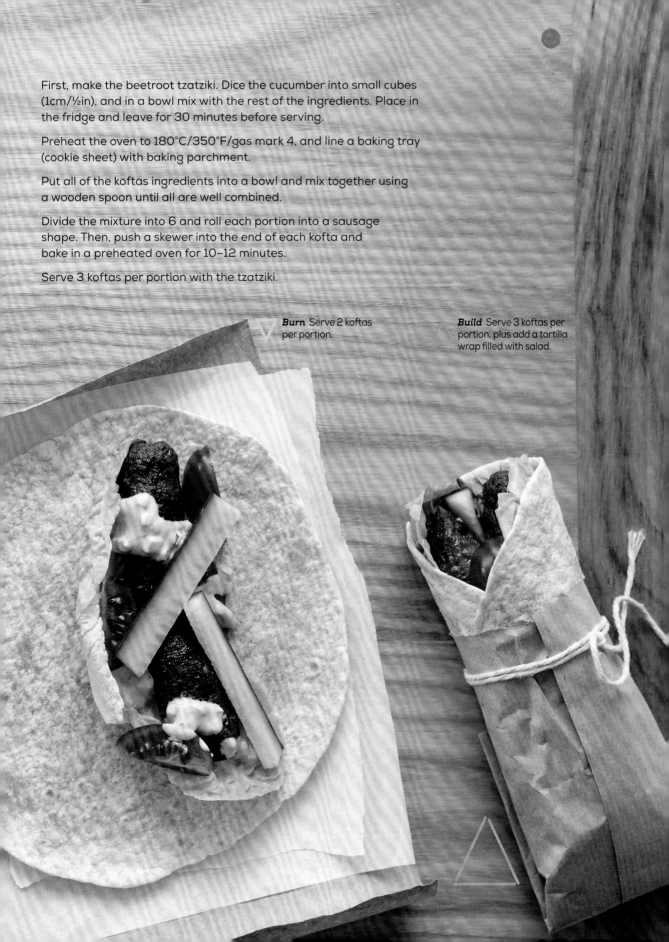

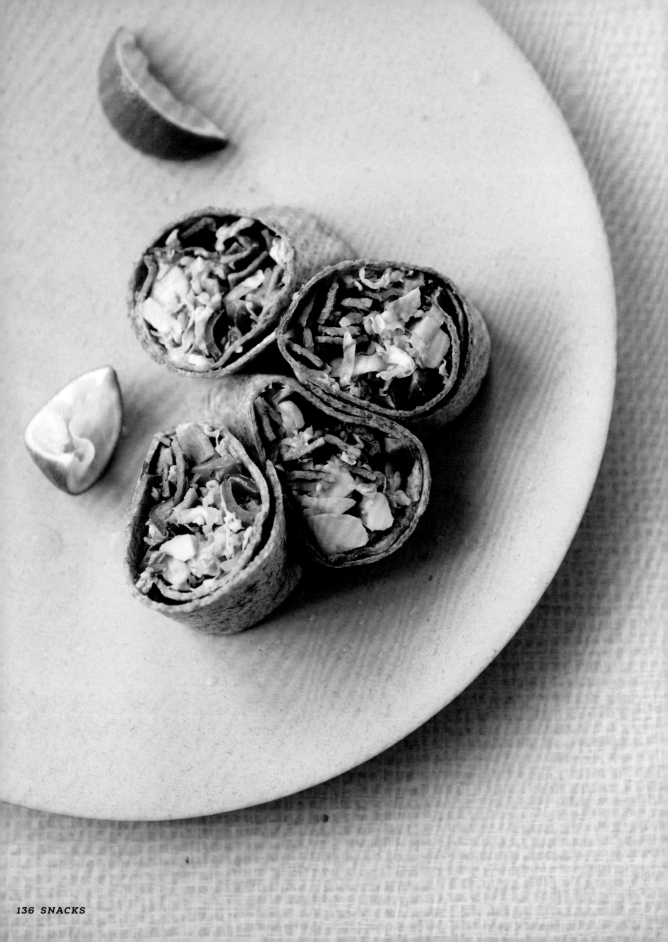

Mini BLT with avocado, lime and chilli

A great twist on the original BLT, the avocado makes it creamy and the chilli and lime give it a zing and a kick to liven up this mini snack.

Health Capsaicin in chillies is a thermogenic compound, which increases the metabolic rate and aids the fat burning process.

Top tip To make this wrap even leaner, try using turkey bacon instead of regular back (Canadian) bacon.

SERVES 2

4 rashers (slices) back (Canadian) bacon

35g (1¼oz) baby gem (Boston) or Cos (romaine) lettuce, shredded

50g (1¾oz) cherry tomatoes, quartered

½ small red chilli, deseeded and finely sliced

finely grated zest and juice of ½ lime

1 wholewheat tortilla

½ avocado, stoned and diced

Preheat the grill (broiler) to a medium high heat. Meanwhile, trim all the fat from the bacon and grill (broil) until browned on both sides. Allow to cool a little and roughly chop into pieces.

Mix together the lettuce, tomatoes, chilli and lime zest in a bowl.

Heat the tortilla under the grill (broiler) for 30 seconds on each side.

Then, simply line up all of the ingredients along the middle of the tortilla and squeeze over the lime juice. Fold 3 edges over and roll up into a burrito-style wrap, cut in half or in quarters and serve.

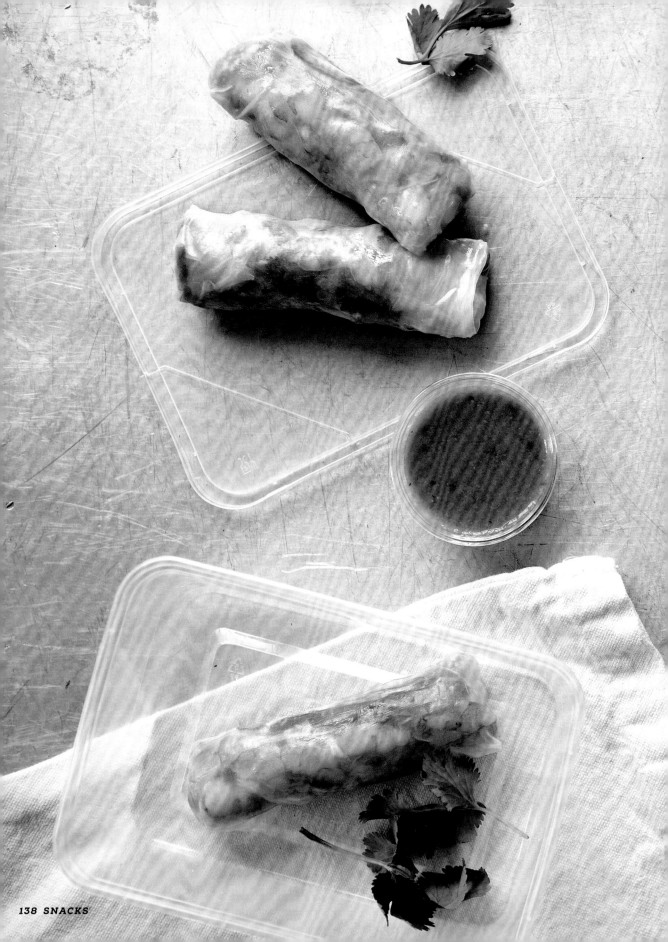

Vietnamese paper rolls with a fragrant sauce

These pretty little rolls are packed with a variety of textures and interesting flavours. A mix of crunchy raw vegetables, fragrant herbs and soft noodles, all stuffed into a light wrapper make a great snack or starter.

Health These rolls are gluten free, low in fat and vitamin-rich! Stuff as many fresh vegetables as you can into a wrapper to make this super-healthy treat.

Top tip For those who like it hot, throw some finely sliced red chilli into the vegetable mix.

SERVES 2

FOR THE FILLING:

70g (2½oz) cooked king prawns (shrimp), pork loin or chicken breast, cut into thin strips

1 small carrot, peeled and grated

3 spring onions (scallions), finely sliced

½ baby gem (Boston) lettuce, shredded

50g (1¾oz) cucumber, peeled and grated

5g (⅛oz) coriander (cilantro) leaves, shredded

6 sheets Vietnamese rice paper wraps, rehydrated

FOR THE SAUCE:

8 lychees, skinned and stoned

1cm (½in) cube root ginger

1cm (½in) piece lemongrass

¼ tsp dried chilli (red pepper) flakes

½ clove garlic

1 tsp honey

½ tsp light soy sauce

juice of ½ lime

First, prepare the ingredients and then divide into 6 equal portions.

Lay each paper wrap on a plate. Add a portion of each ingredient to the middle of each wrap and roll these up into a mini burrito-style wrap.

Then, make the sauce. Using a beaker and hand-held blender, blitz all of the ingredients until smooth. Transfer into a ramekin or shallow dish.

Serve 3 paper rolls per portion with the dipping sauce.

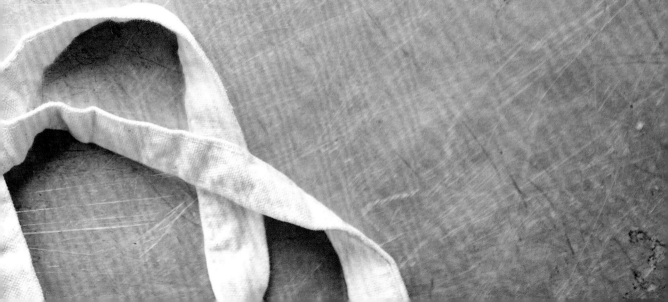

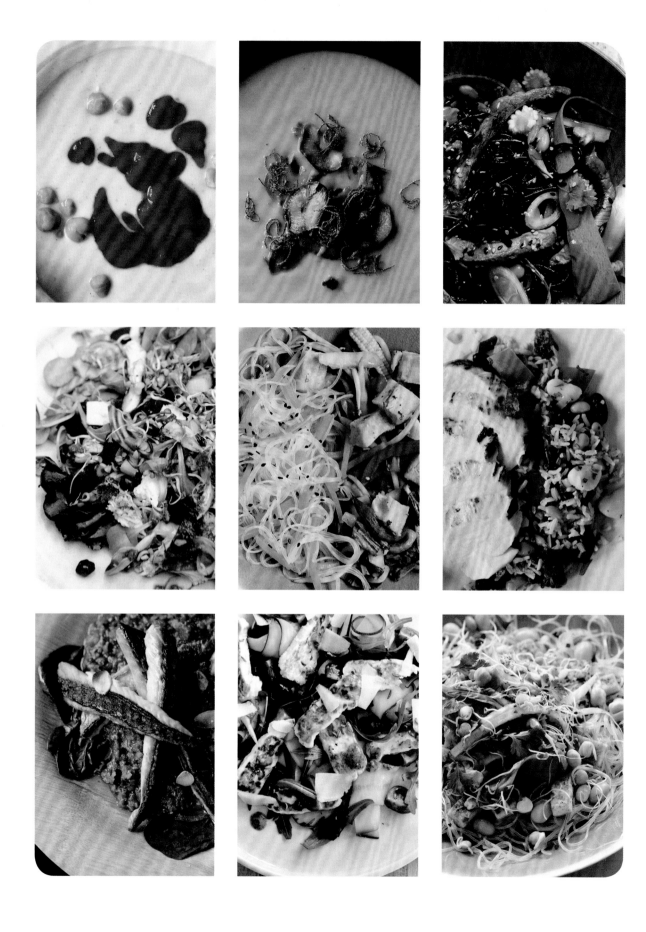

MAIN MEALS

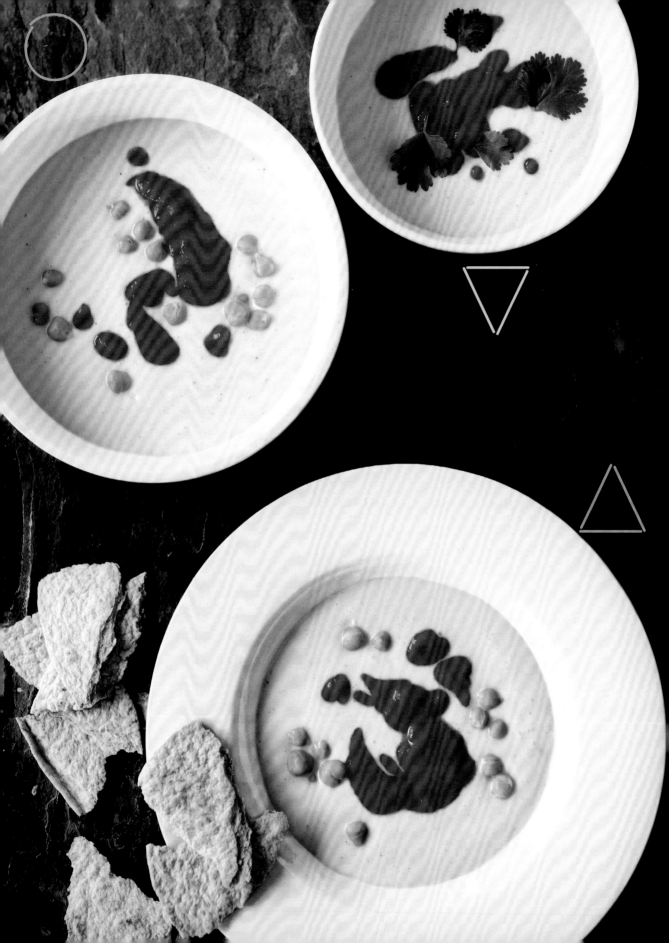

Moroccan-spiced pepper and cauliflower soup

The combination of roasted peppers and cauliflower mixed with a Moroccan spice blend and harissa make this power-packed vegetable soup irresistible.

Health Red (bell) peppers are one of the best sources of vitamin C, which can help maintain immunity as well as acting as a potent antioxidant.

Top tip This soup freezes well, so make a large batch and pop in the freezer for a quick lunch to take to work or to grab at the weekend.

SERVES 2

3 red (bell) peppers

1 small cauliflower, sliced

¼ onion, sliced

1 clove garlic, roughly chopped

¼ tsp ground cinnamon

½ tsp ground allspice

2.5g organic vegetable bouillon (¼ cube or ¾ tsp powder)

800ml (3½ cups) whole milk

1 tsp harissa paste

sea salt and freshly ground black pepper

Preheat the oven to 200°C/400°F/gas mark 6, and you'll need a baking tray (cookie sheet).

Slice the red flesh from the (bell) peppers, discarding the stalk and seeded parts. On a baking tray (cookie sheet) in a preheated oven, roast the peppers for 10–15 minutes until soft.

Put the cauliflower, onion and garlic along with the cinnamon, allspice, bouillon and the milk into a large pan with a lid and bring to the boil. Reduce to a simmer and cook until the cauliflower is soft.

Remove the peppers from the oven and transfer to a blender along with the harissa and blitz until smooth. Season to taste and set aside.

Rinse the blender and transfer the cauliflower mixture from the pan to the blender and blitz till smooth. Add more milk if necessary to create the desired consistency. Season to taste.

To serve, gently reheat both the cauliflower soup and the pepper purée in separate pans. Pour the cauliflower soup into 2 bowls and add a few tablespoons of the pepper purée to the centre of each bowl.

Balance At the end add 40g (¼ cup) cooked chickpeas per portion to the soup.

Build As well as adding the chickpeas (see left), help yourself to some pitta crisps. Tear half a wholemeal (wholewheat) pitta (per portion) into pieces and bake in the oven (at 120°C/250°F/gas mark ½) until crispy.

Celeriac, vanilla and tarragon soup

A warm, hearty bowl of soup is all you need when it's cold outside! Celeriac is in season from September to April, and here this nobbly vegetable is matched beautifully with aromatic vanilla and tarragon.

Health This soup is jam-packed with antibacterial properties due to the garlic, ginger and onion – perfect for keeping colds at bay.

Sport The celeriac provides a beneficial amount of vitamin K. In addition, there's a good hit of calcium in the milk for keeping bones strong.

SERVES 2

¼ onion, chopped

1 celeriac (about 600g/1lb 5oz in weight), chopped

1 garlic clove, finely chopped

1cm (½ in) piece root ginger, finely chopped

seeds from 1 vanilla pod (bean)

1 tsp black mustard seeds

700ml (3 cups) skimmed milk

½ tsp organic vegetable bouillon powder

sea salt, to taste

2–3 sprigs tarragon, plus extra to garnish (optional)

Add all the ingredients (except the salt and tarragon) to a pan with a lid. Cover and bring to the boil. Then, simmer until the celeriac is soft.

Transfer the contents of the pan to a blender and blitz until smooth, adding more milk if necessary. Season with salt, to taste.

Pick the leaves from the tarragon, add to the soup and blitz again for 10–15 seconds. To serve, gently reheat and divide between 2 bowls and garnish with a few more tarragon leaves.

Super-green pearl barley soup

Fuel any outdoor activities with this warming soup. Its combination of slow-release, complex carbohydrates will keep you going for longer.

Health As well as providing a slow-release form of energy, this super-green soup has plenty of micronutrients to support your body's immunity.

Sport Liquid diets can be useful for athletes who need to pile on weight or drop weight quickly. This soup allows you to eat the calories and gain nutrients.

SERVES 4

½ medium carrot, diced

¼ medium sweet potato, diced

½ small onion, diced

1 stick celery, diced

1 tsp vegetable oil

1.3 litres (5½ cups) water, plus an extra 100ml (scant ½ cup) for thickening if necessary

10g (⅓oz) organic vegetable bouillon (1 cube or 3 tsp powder)

2½ tsp thyme leaves, picked

1½ tsp roasted garlic paste (see page 106)

80g (⅓ cup) pearl barley

2 tsp cornflour (cornstarch)

200g (7oz) spinach

salt and white pepper, to taste

Place the carrot, sweet potato, onion and celery into a large pan on a medium heat. Then, add the oil and, when hot, cook the vegetables for 6–8 minutes until starting to soften.

Add the water, bouillon, thyme, garlic and pearl barley and bring to the boil. Reduce to a simmer and cook for 30–40 minutes until the vegetables and barley are soft.

Remove from the heat and allow to cool a little. Transfer to a blender and blitz until smooth. Return to the pan and bring back to the boil. If the soup needs thickening mix the cornflour (cornstarch) and 100ml (scant ½ cup) of water together in a cup and mix into the soup a little at a time, stirring constantly.

Put 50g (1¾oz) of the spinach into a blender and blitz, add 50g (1¾oz) more at a time and continue to blitz until all the spinach has been puréed. Add this purée to the soup and season. Serve straightaway.

If you are making this soup in advance, don't add the spinach purée until you are just about to serve it, otherwise the vibrant green colour will be lost.

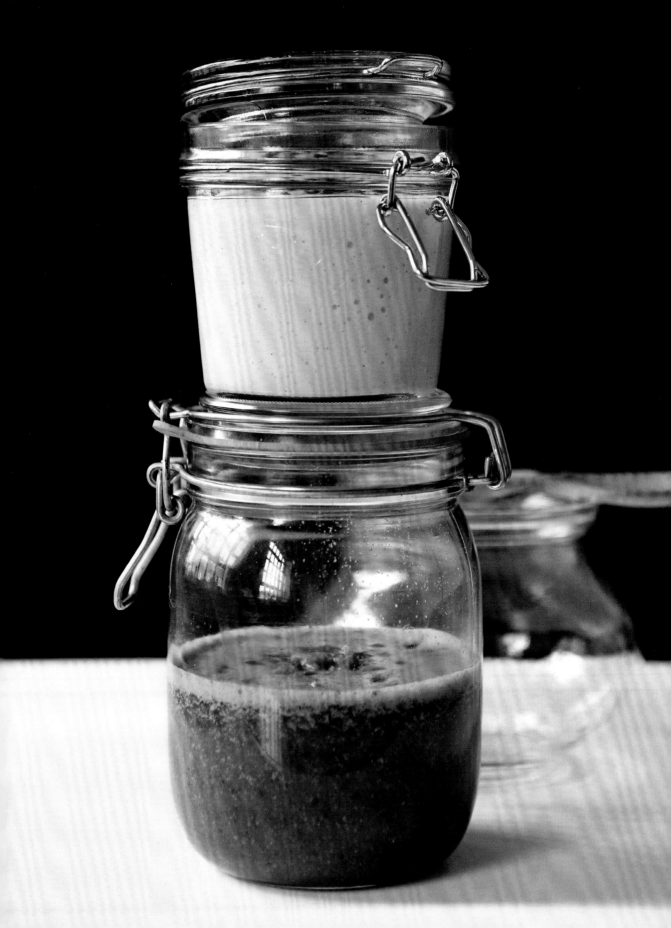

Clear tomato and coconut soup

While it may not be one of the quickest of dishes to make, it's certainly worth the wait. This refreshing soup is ideally served chilled on a summer evening.

Sport The coconut water has great levels of electrolytes that are essential for maintaining and replenishing hydration levels pre- or post-training.

Top tip You can make the tomato water in large batches to freeze if you find a box of over-ripe tomatoes at your local greengrocer being sold off cheap. This tomato water also makes a great alternative in smoothies and Virgin Bloody Marys.

SERVES 2

30g (½ cup) coriander (cilantro) leaves, plus extra to garnish
20g (1 cup) flat-leaf parsley
2cm (¾in) piece lemongrass
1.5kg (3lb 5oz) very ripe tomatoes
1 tsp sea salt
250ml (1 cup) coconut water
60g (2¼oz) edamame

Put the coriander (cilantro), parsley and lemongrass into a large bowl and sit a colander on top. Wet a 1-metre (30-in) long piece of muslin (cheesecloth), squeeze the excess water out and fold it in half and sit it on top of the colander.

Set aside 1 tomato and then remove the stalks from the rest of tomatoes, quarter each one and place onto the muslin (cheesecloth) in the colander. Sprinkle the salt on top of the tomatoes and fold the edges of the muslin (cheesecloth) over to cover. Transfer the bowl and colander to the fridge for 24 hours (you may need to make some room).

The next day, remove from the fridge and strain the herbs and tomato water through a fine sieve (strainer) into a large jug (pitcher).

Add the coconut water and a little more salt, to taste.

Peel the skin off the reserved tomato and cut into thin strips and set aside. Split the edamame between 2 bowls, pour on the chilled soup and garnish with a few coriander (cilantro) leaves and the tomato skin strips.

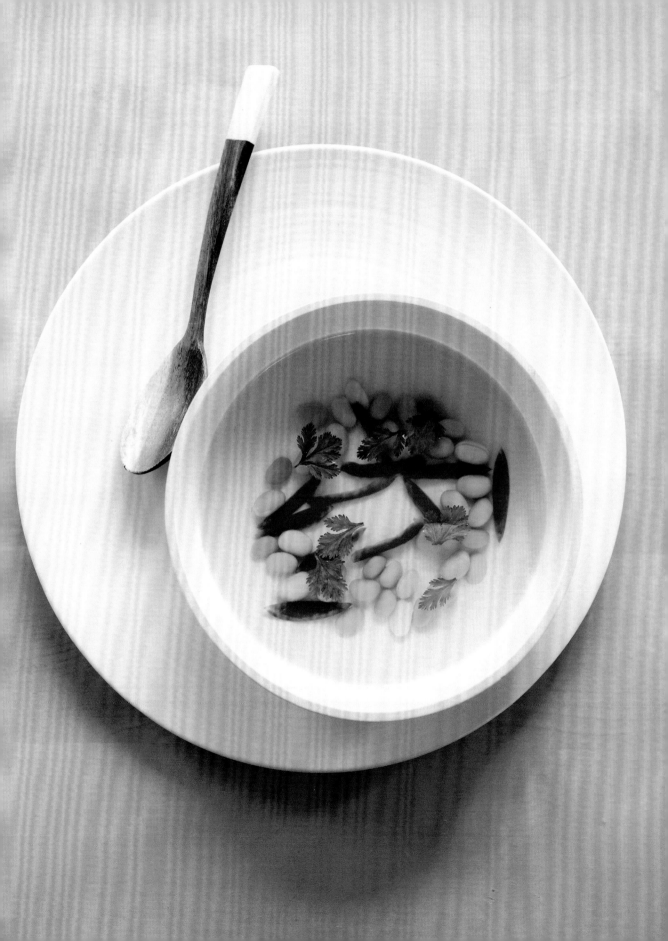

Butternut squash, sage and chestnut soup

With its thick and creamy texture, this soup is sure to become a real crowd pleaser. The sweetness of the butternut squash creates a pleasing contrast to the deep, earthy flavour of sage.

Health Butternut squash and chestnuts are good sources of vitamin C and manganese. The vitamin B6 in the squash is vital for haemoglobin formation.

Sport Quark is a very low-fat, high-protein cheese, so it gives this soup a super-shot of protein.

SERVES 2

1 butternut squash (about 800g/1lb 12oz in weight), peeled, deseeded and cut into small pieces
500ml (2 cups) water
2 tsp organic vegetable bouillon powder
50g (scant ¼ cup) quark or crème fraîche
sea salt, to taste
1 tsp chopped sage leaves
3 tsp chopped sweet chestnuts (we use vacuum-packed ones)

Place the squash pieces along with half of the water and all of the bouillon into a pan with a lid, and bring to the boil. Reduce the heat to a simmer and continue to cook until the squash is soft.

Transfer the contents of the pan to a blender along with the quark (or crème fraîche) and blitz until smooth, adding more water as necessary. Season with salt, to taste.

Return the soup to the pan and reheat to a simmer. Pour half into each of 2 bowls and top with the sage and chestnuts.

Thai beetroot soup

This eye-catching soup is so simple to make but tastes delicious. Warm yourself up on a chilly day with this vibrant and nutritious soup.

Health The electrolytes found in coconut milk can help maintain hydration during the day.

Sport Beetroot is a great source of dietary nitrates, which helps your body perform better on the same amount of oxygen.

SERVES 2

350g (12oz) cooked beetroot
10g (⅓oz) organic vegetable bouillon (1 cube or 3 tsp powder)
2 tsp Thai red curry paste
300ml (1¼ cups) water
220ml (1 cup) coconut milk
sea salt, to taste
coriander (cilantro) leaves, to garnish

In a blender, blitz the beetroot, bouillon, curry paste and water until smooth. Pour into a pan and add 200ml (scant 1 cup) of the coconut milk, stirring well. Bring to the boil and add salt, to taste.

To serve, pour between 2 bowls and garnish with swirls of the remaining coconut milk and the coriander (cilantro).

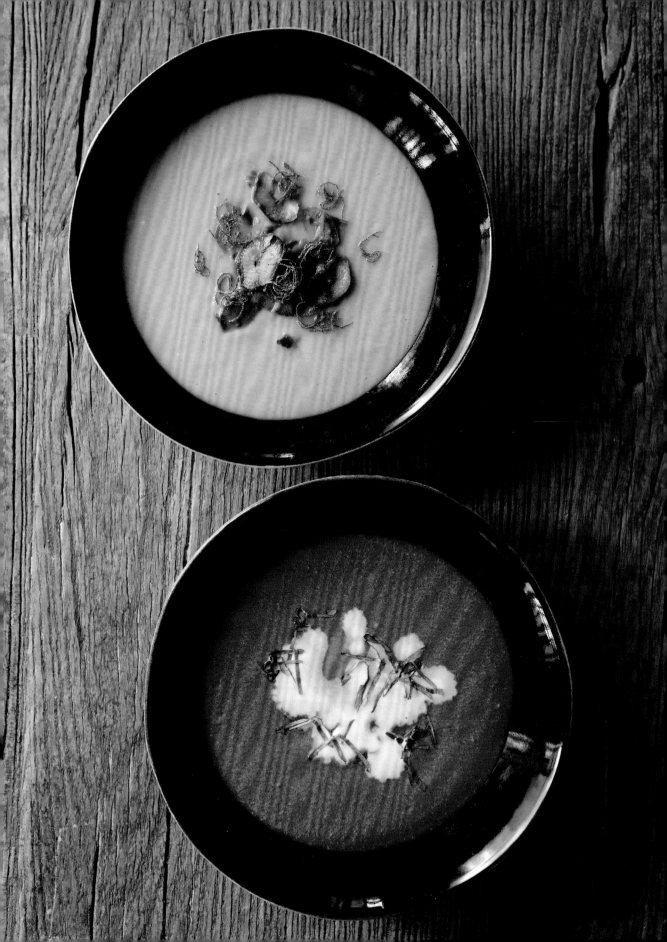

Chicken with giant couscous, fennel, pear and walnuts

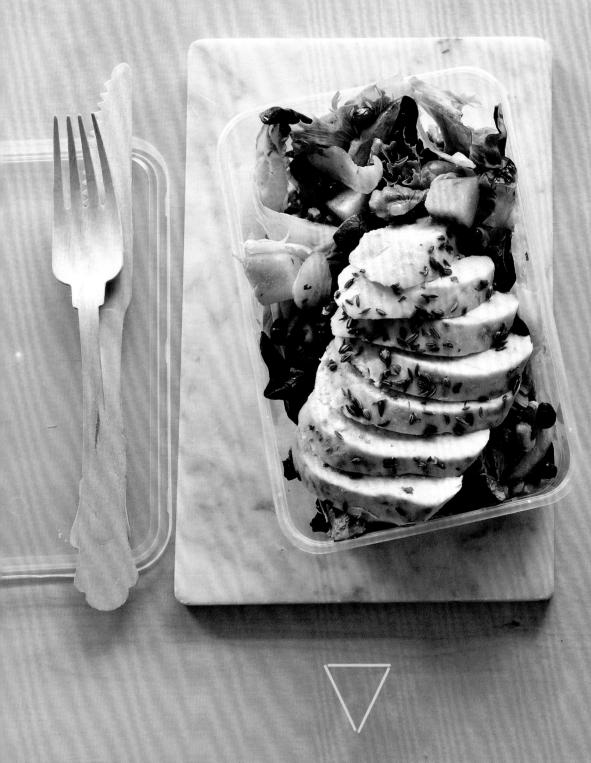

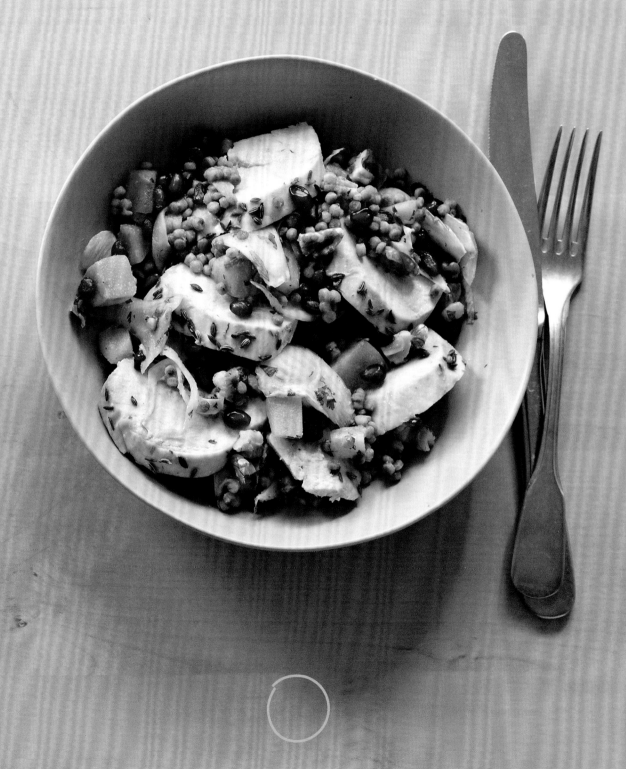

Chicken with giant couscous, fennel, pear and walnuts

A really fresh and fruity dish that leaves you feeling very satisfied without being too heavy.

Health The pears contain high levels of pectin (a water-soluble fibre) that can aid digestion and regulate blood sugar.

Sport The antioxidants in the pomegranates help to counter any muscle soreness.

SERVES 2

2 chicken breasts (a total weight of 240–280g/8½–10oz)

¾ tsp fennel seeds

½ tsp cumin seeds

a pinch of salt, plus extra to taste

100g (½ cup) giant couscous

2 large bulbs of fennel (about 160g/5½oz in total weight)

3 Conference pears (about 150g/5½oz in total weight)

1 pomegranate

1 sprig flat-leaf parsley

1 sprig coriander (cilantro)

50g (½ cup) walnuts, crushed

finely grated zest of ½ lemon

15g (1 tbsp) honey

Preheat the oven to 190°C/375°F/gas mark 5, and you'll need 2 baking trays (cookie sheets).

Place the chicken onto a baking tray (cookie sheet) and sprinkle with the fennel seeds, cumin seeds and the salt. Bake in the preheated oven for 15 minutes until cooked through (if you have a meat probe the core temperature should be 65°C/149°F).

Cook the couscous according to the packet instructions, as the large couscous does vary in size so the cooking times can be quite different.

Slice the fennel bulbs as thinly as you can – I like to use a Japanese mandolin – trying not to include any of the harder root section.

Peel and core the pears then chop into small chunks and place along with the fennel onto a baking tray (cookie sheet) and bake for 10–12 minutes.

Cut the pomegranate in half and remove the seeds. To do this, hold one half with the cut side over a bowl and firmly tap the back of it with a rolling pin until all the seeds fall out; repeat with the other half. Pick the leaves from the herbs and slice them finely.

Take one-third of the baked pear pieces and, using the back of a fork in a small bowl, crush into a rough purée.

In a large bowl, mix together the couscous, pear, pear purée, fennel, walnuts, lemon zest, half of the herbs, half of the pomegranate seeds and add a little salt, if necessary, to taste. To serve, divide between 2 bowls, top with the chicken breast and sprinkle over the rest of the herbs and pomegranate seeds.

Burn Remove the couscous from the recipe and add 130g (4½oz) per portion of diced celeriac. Roast the celeriac along with the fennel and pear.

Build Simply add an extra 30g (scant ¼ cup) couscous per portion.

Pesto and crème fraîche chicken

This super-speedy, easy peasy dish is perfect for those evenings when you don't have a lot of time but you still want something nutritious and delicious for dinner.

Health An all-round, well-balanced dish that's packed with lots of vegetables to give your immune system a boost.

Top tip This dish is so versatile! Swap in your favourite vegetables. Why not try adding sunblush tomatoes, Pepperdew, courgettes or aubergines.

SERVES 2

- 120g (4½oz) sweet potato, diced
- 2 chicken breast (a total weight of 240g/8½oz), cubed
- 2 tsp extra virgin olive oil
- ½ small red onion, chopped
- 70g (2½oz) chestnut (cremini) mushrooms, quartered
- 60g (2¼oz) baby corn, sliced
- 1 clove garlic, chopped
- 60g (2¼oz) asparagus tips
- 100g (3½oz) baby plum tomatoes
- 200g (scant 1 cup) low-fat crème fraîche

FOR THE PESTO:

- 30g (1 cup) basil leaves, shredded
- 25g (¼ cup) pine nuts
- 15g (1 tbsp) Parmesan cheese, grated
- sea salt and freshly ground black pepper to taste

First, make the pesto. Using a blender, blitz the basil leaves, pine nuts and grated Parmesan together to make a smooth paste. Season with salt and pepper to taste.

Cook the sweet potato in a pan of boiling water until cooked but still firm.

Meanwhile, place the chicken and 1 teaspoon of the oil into a hot frying pan (skillet) over a medium heat until cooked (break a piece in half or check with a needle probe, it should read 65°C/149°F). Tip the chicken pieces into a bowl and return the pan to the heat and turn it up to high.

Add the remaining oil to the pan along with the onion, mushrooms, baby corn and garlic and cook for 2 minutes, then add the asparagus and cook for a further 2 minutes.

Next, add the pesto and the rest of the ingredients and fold together, cook through until piping hot and then season to taste. Divide into 2 and serve straightaway.

▽ **Burn** Replace the sweet potato with the same weight per portion of carrot and cook along with the rest of the vegetables.

△ **Build** Cook a 'nest' of spinach tagliatelle pasta per portion and add this to the rest of the ingredients at the end.

Pesto and crème fraîche chicken

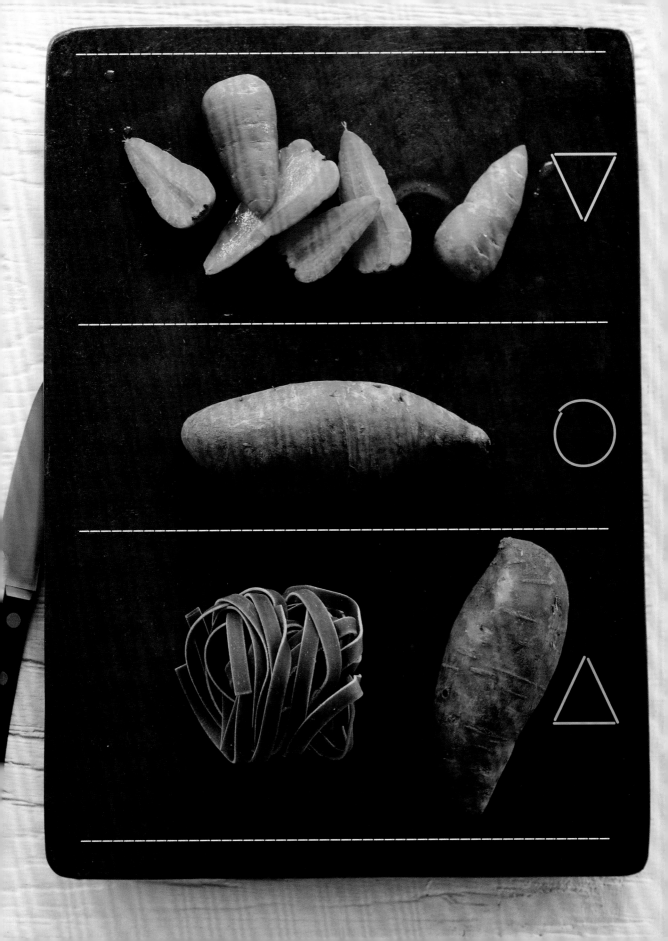

Sesame black noodles with soy and ginger duck

This Asian-inspired dish is an impressive one to serve up to friends and family. The tastes are amazingly fresh with a satisfying crunch, too.

Health Ginger is a potent antibacterial agent and so is great for maintaining immunity.

Sport This dish is high in vitamin B12, which can help prevent megaloblastic anaemia – a condition that would reduce a person's endurance capacity.

SERVES 4

- 60g (2¼oz) carrots
- 100g (3½oz) asparagus
- 10g (⅓oz) red chilli
- 40g (1½oz) spring onions (scallions)
- 40g (1½oz) baby corn
- 85g (3¼oz) raw black rice noodles (340g/12oz) cooked weight)
- 1 tsp coconut or rapeseed (canola) oil, for stir-frying
- 200g (7oz) duck breast, cut into strips
- 40g (1½oz) baby leaf spinach
- 40g (1½oz) edamame
- 85g (3¼oz) sugar snap peas
- 5g (⅙oz) mixed white and black sesame seeds
- 5g (⅙oz) mint leaves, picked
- 10g (⅓oz) pickled ginger, cut into matchsticks
- 40g (¼ cup) cashew nuts

FOR THE GINGER AND SOY DRESSING (MAKES A JAR FULL):

- 85g (3¼oz) stem (preserved) ginger in syrup
- 5 tbsp lemon juice
- a thumb of fresh root ginger, peeled
- 5 tbsp soy sauce
- 150ml (⅔ cup) extra virgin olive oil

Using a vegetable peeler, peel the carrots and then once peeled use the peeler to make carrot 'ribbons', allowing them to fall into a large bowl.

Take the woody bottoms off the asparagus and, again using a peeler, turn into asparagus ribbons, adding to the bowl as before.

Slice the red chilli on an angle and do the same with the spring onions (scallions) and baby corn and pop into the large bowl.

Make the dressing. Blitz the stem (preserved) ginger with the lemon juice and pass through a sieve (strainer); if you don't have a high-speed blender then grate the ginger first. Next, add the soy sauce and oil and mix together. Set aside. (The dressing recipe makes more than you need so freeze the leftovers in ice cube trays and then, in future, defrost one ice cube for enough salad dressing for this recipe.)

Bring a pan of water to the boil and cook the noodles for 8 minutes. Meanwhile, start to cook the duck. Add the oil to a large frying pan (skillet) or wok and stir-fry the duck for 2 minutes.

When the noodles are cooked, drain and mix with the prepared vegetables and add the other ingredients, with 1 tablespoon of the dressing going on last. Mix well together and divide between four bowls and top with the cooked duck.

▽ **Burn** Follow the above recipe, but instead of using black rice noodles make courgette (zucchini) 'noodles'. Take 50g (1¾oz) courgettes (zucchini) and spiralise them using a Japanese vegetable turning machine (mouli) or a spiraliser; you can buy them at all good cook shops.

△ **Build** Follow the above recipe, but finish off with an extra topping of roasted sweet potato and cashews per portion. So, before you start the above recipe, preheat the oven to 200°C/ 400°F/gas mark 6. Roast 50g (1¾oz) sweet potato, cut into cubes and tossed in a little sunflower oil for 20 minutes. Mix with 20g (scant ¼ cup) cashew nuts and scatter on top.

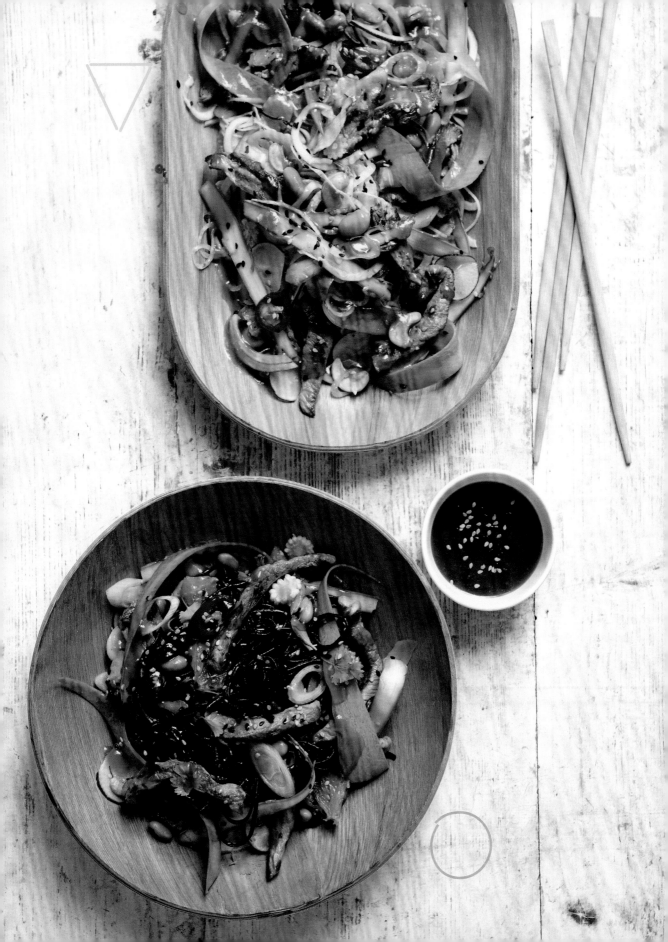

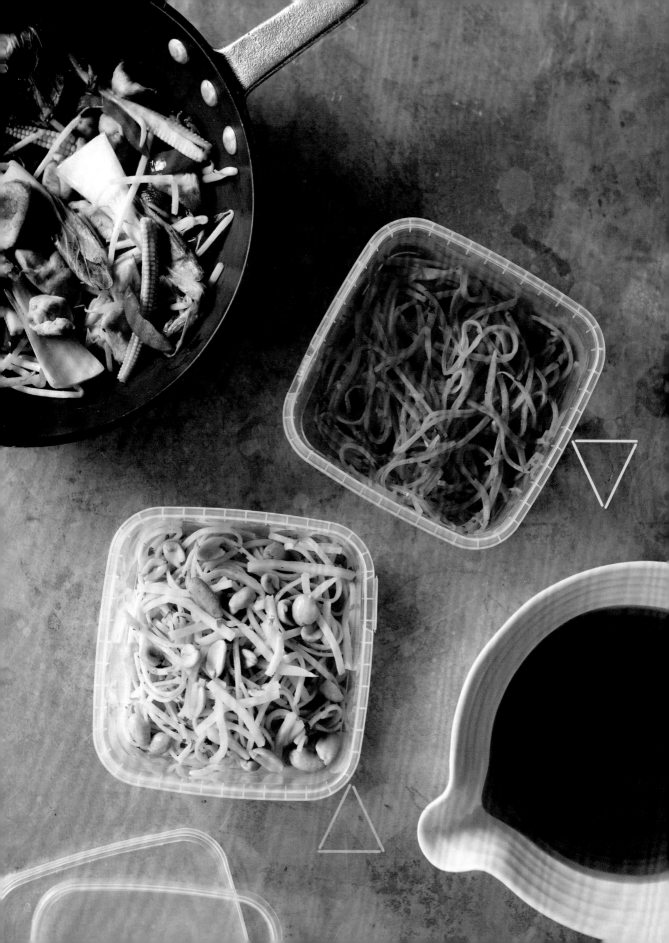

Chilli chicken ramen

This oriental-inspired fragrant and sharp dish is packed full of flavour and nutrients. It's an easy one-pot dish as you just throw everything in and let the fresh aromas infuse the light stock.

Health Immunity is the key emphasis of this dish as it's packed full of antibacterial properties from the ginger, chilli and garlic.

Top tip Why not make a large batch and keep half refrigerated for a couple of days; the taste improves with time as well!

SERVES 2

2 chicken breasts (a total weight of 240–280g/8½–10oz)

1 red (bell) pepper

1 pak choi

80g (3¼oz) shiitake mushrooms

60g (2¼oz) baby corn

½ red chilli, deseeded

1 tsp sesame oil

40g (scant ½ cup) beansprouts

100g (3½oz) wholewheat egg noodles

FOR THE BROTH:

670ml (3 cups) water

15g (½oz) organic chicken bouillon (1½ cubes)

8g lemongrass, chopped

2cm (¾in) cube root ginger, peeled and chopped

1 medium-sized red chilli, deseeded and chopped

2 cloves garlic, chopped

3 salad tomatoes, quartered

40g (scant 1 cup) coriander (cilantro), chopped, plus extra to garnish

2½ tbsp fish sauce

6 mint leaves

4 spring onions (scallions), chopped

12g (5 tsp) palm sugar

juice of 1 lime

First, make the broth. Put all the ingredients into a pan and bring to the boil, reduce to a simmer and cook for 20 minutes. Remove from the heat and allow the flavours to infuse for a further 20 minutes, then strain through a sieve (strainer) into a large pan.

Preheat the oven to 180°C/350°F/gas mark 4, and you'll need a baking tray (cookie sheet).

In a hot frying pan (skillet) or on a griddle, colour the chicken on one side (no oil is needed). Place on the baking tray (cookie sheet) browned side up and bake in a preheated oven for 15 minutes until cooked (if you have a meat probe the core temperature should be 65°C/149°F). Remove from the oven and slice.

Reheat the broth and bring it to a boil. Meanwhile, thinly slice the pepper, pak choi, mushrooms, baby corn and chilli. Add the oil to a hot frying pan (skillet) then the sliced vegetables followed by the beansprouts and cook for 2–3 minutes over a high heat.

Next, cook the noodles according to the packet instructions and, when cooked, drain in a colander. To serve, divide the hot broth between 2 large bowls, share out the vegetables and noodles, top with the sliced chicken and garnish with some chopped coriander (cilantro).

▽ **Burn** Replace the egg noodles with mooli (daikon) 'noodles'. Take 120g (4½oz) mooli (daikon) per portion and using a Japanese vegetable turner or spiraliser transform them into noodles. Steam for 3–4 minutes.

△ **Build** Throw in 15g (scant ⅛ cup) cashew nuts and an extra 25g (1oz) noodles per portion.

Keralan rasam

Rasam is a great dish as it's so versatile – it can be served as a soup or as a curry with rice. Whichever way you serve it, the spices warm you from the inside out!

Health Almonds are packed with vitamin E to help protect cell membranes and cell structure.

Sport Full of antioxidant-crammed spices and ingredients, this nutritious dish can help fight the increased oxidative stress from heavy exercise.

SERVES 2

½ tsp black mustard seeds
seeds of 4 cardamom pods
½ tsp fennel seeds
1 tsp ground cumin
2 tsp ground coriander
½ tsp nutmeg
2 cloves
¼ tsp flaked chilli
2 cloves garlic
1cm (½in) cube root ginger
200ml (scant 1 cup) tinned low-fat coconut milk
300ml (1¼ cups) almond milk
½ tsp tamarind paste
30g (¼ cup) goji berries
30g (⅓ cup) ground almonds
1 small sweet potato (about 150g/5½oz in weight), diced
1 parsnip, diced
2 chicken breasts (a total of weight of 280g/10oz)
1 banana, sliced
70g (2½oz) spinach leaves, shredded
6g (⅛oz) coriander (cilantro) leaves, chopped
1 red chilli, sliced to garnish (optional)

Preheat the oven to 180°C/350°F/gas mark 4.

In a dry frying pan (skillet) over a low heat add the spices and dry toast for 2–3 minutes. Next, empty these into a beaker, add the garlic, ginger and half of the coconut milk and blitz with a hand-held blender until quite smooth (about 1–1½ minutes). Put this sauce along with the rest of the coconut milk, almond milk, tamarind paste, goji berries and ground almonds into a large pan and bring to the boil. Then, reduce the heat to a simmer. Next, add the sweet potato and parsnip to the sauce and cook for 6–8 minutes.

In a hot frying pan (skillet) or on a griddle, colour the chicken on one side (no oil is needed). Place on the baking tray (cookie sheet) browned side up and bake in a preheated oven for 15 minutes until cooked (if you have a meat probe the core temperature should be 65°C/149°F). Remove from the oven and slice.

Add the banana to the sauce and continue to cook until the vegetables soften; add more almond milk, if necessary. About 2–3 minutes before the end of its cooking time, fold in the spinach. To serve, divide the vegetables and sauce between 2 bowls, top with the chicken and garnish with the chopped coriander (cilantro) and chilli, if required.

Burn Replace the sweet potato with 80g (⅔ cup) diced courgette (zucchini) per portion and add this to the pan along with the parsnips.

 Build Give yourself a 50g (1¾oz) portion of rice or have a chapatti with the meal.

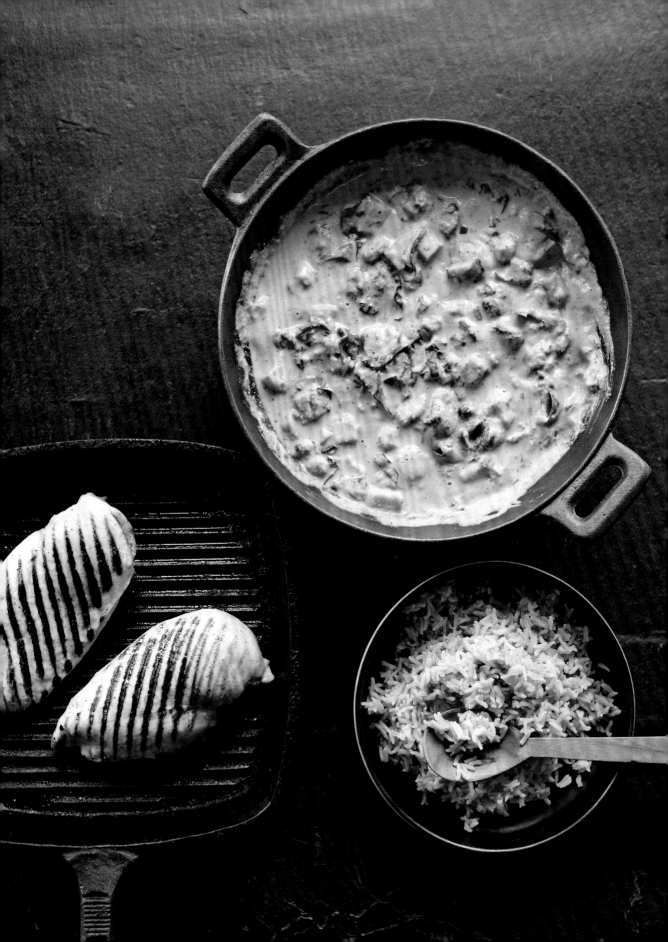

Saffron-poached chicken, barberry rice and baba ganoush

This fragrant Middle Eastern slow-cooked dish combines heat, aroma and an array of textures, culminating in a total feast for the senses.

Health Persian barberries have many beneficial properties, including lowering blood pressure and acting as an anti-inflammatory.

Top tip Pair brown rice with other lean proteins such as chicken or fish. To make it more flavoursome, use a chicken stock instead of the cooking water.

SERVES 2

4 skinless, boneless chicken thighs (a total weight of 350g/12oz)

400ml (1¾ cups) water

5g (⅙oz) organic chicken bouillon (½ cube)

½ star anise

4 bay leaves

25 strands saffron

2 cloves garlic

sea salt and freshly ground black pepper

1 aubergine (eggplant), halved

2½ tsp extra virgin olive oil

¾ tsp roasted garlic paste (see page 106)

1½ tsp tahini

1 tbsp chopped flat-leaf parsley

juice of ¼ lemon

1 tsp harissa paste

80g (scant ⅓ cup) Greek yogurt

100g (½ cup) brown basmati rice

20g (¾oz) barberries

¼ red onion, finely chopped

½ courgette (zucchini) (about 100g/3½oz), diced

80g (3¼oz) cherry tomatoes, halved

½ clove garlic, chopped

20g (¾oz) rocket (arugula)

Preheat the oven to 140°C/275°F/gas mark 1, and you'll need a 2-litre (2-quart) ovenproof dish with a lid and a baking tray (cookie sheet).

Place the chicken, water, bouillon, star anise, bay leaves and saffron in the ovenproof dish. Crush the garlic cloves and add these along with a pinch of salt. Cover and place in a preheated oven for 3 hours, until the thighs are tender but not falling apart.

Meanwhile, place the aubergine (eggplant) halves onto a baking tray (cookie sheet) cut sides up. Drizzle ½ teaspoon of oil and a pinch of salt over each and bake in the oven for 35–40 minutes. When done, remove from the oven and, using a spoon, scoop out the flesh and place in a bowl. Add ½ teaspoon of the roasted garlic paste and 1 teaspoon of oil along with the tahini, chopped parsley and lemon juice and crush this mixture together using a fork. Season the baba ganoush to taste.

Mix the harissa and remaining garlic paste with the yogurt in a bowl and set aside in the fridge.

Cook the rice in a large pan of boiling water for 20–25 minutes. Five minutes before you think the rice is done, add the barberries to the pan. When cooked, drain well through a sieve (strainer) and return to the pan, fold in the red onion and add a pinch of salt.

In a hot frying pan (skillet) over a high heat add the remaining oil along with the courgette (zucchini). Cook for 2 minutes then add the tomatoes, garlic and rocket (arugula). Cook for a further minute, season with salt, to taste, and serve. To serve, divide the poached chicken between 2 bowls, serving each with half of the rice, courgettes (zucchini), spiced yogurt and baba ganoush.

▽ **Burn** Use a portion of cauliflower 'couscous' (see page 184) in place of the rice here. Add the barberries with the cauliflower, drain then fold in the onion and season.

△ **Build** Either increase the rice serving by a third for each portion or enjoy the meal with a wholemeal (wholewheat) pitta or flatbread.

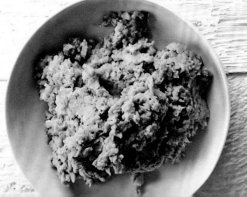

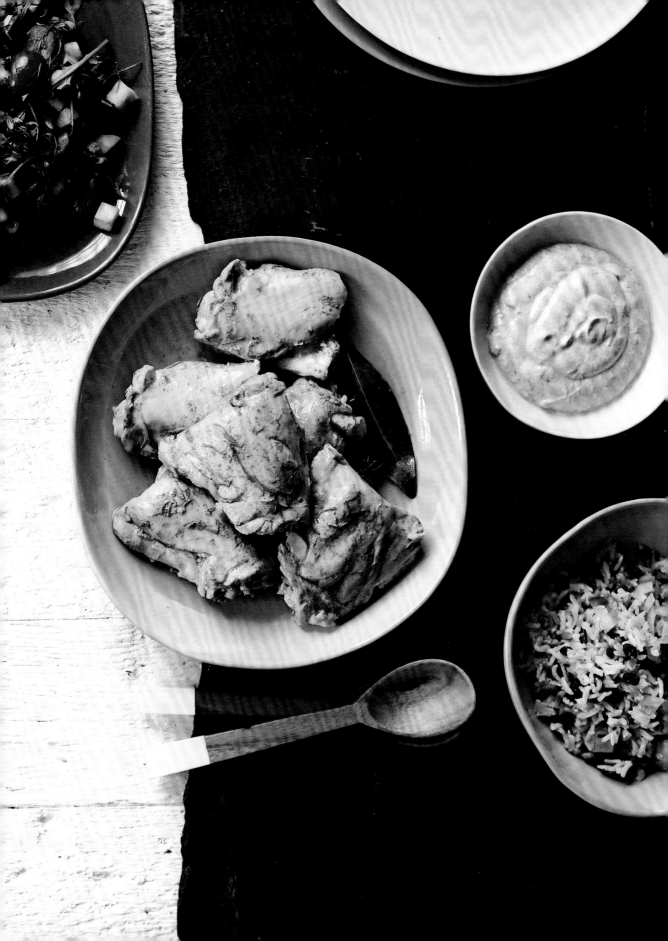

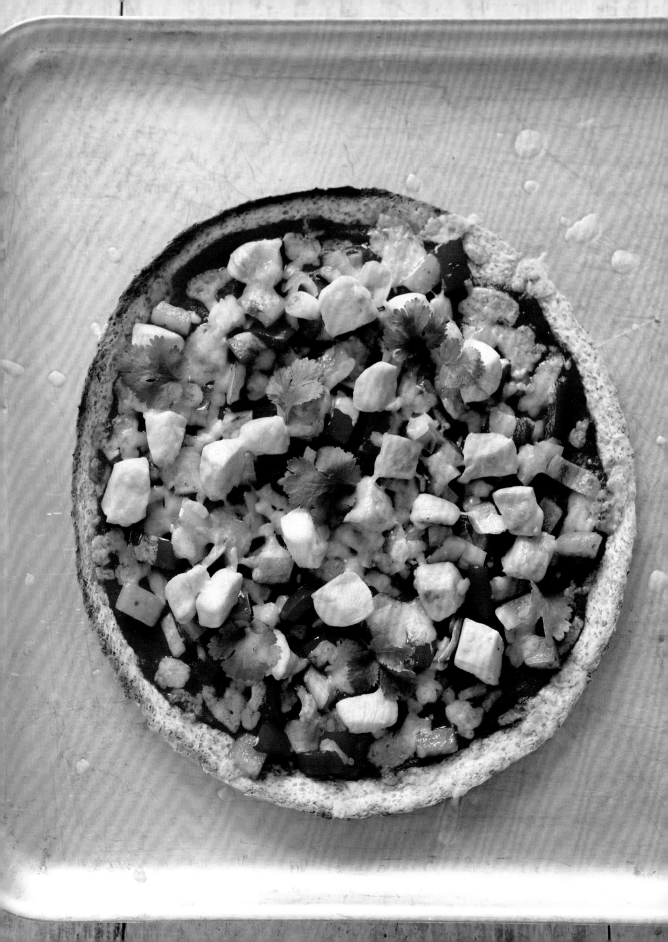

Chicken fajita pizza

This quick and easy meal makes a perfect lunch with a fabulous balance of proteins, fats and complex carbohydrates. It can be eaten hot or cold, so can be made to suit whatever you need.

Health Being topped with plenty of vegetables, this pizza will not only satisfy the taste buds but provide you with two servings of vegetables.

Top tip Having friends over to watch the game? Roll out this healthy pizza to win over fans but without the excess calories.

SERVES 2

2 chicken breasts (a total weight of 240–280g/ 8½–10oz)

2 tsp vegetable oil, for frying

20g (½ cup) coriander (cilantro), chopped

sea salt and cracked black pepper

1 small red onion, thinly sliced

1 small red (bell) pepper or ½ a large pepper, thinly sliced

1 small yellow (bell) pepper or ½ a large pepper, thinly sliced

1 fresh chilli, deseeded and thinly sliced

2 large wholewheat tortilla wraps

60g (½ cup) Cheddar cheese, grated

FOR THE SAUCE:

½ onion

½ clove garlic

1 tsp vegetable oil, for frying

400g (14oz) tin chopped tomatoes

10g (1½ tsp) agave syrup

2 tbsp tomato purée (paste)

1 tsp fajita seasoning

First make the pizza sauce. Finely dice the onion and roughly chop or crush the garlic and place in a medium sized pan with the oil, on a medium heat cook the onions and garlic until soft – you don't want any colour on them.

Next, add the tomatoes, agave syrup, tomato purée (paste) and fajita seasoning and bring to the boil and simmer. Cook until it has reduced down to half its original volume. Allow to cool a little and then pour into a blender (or use a hand-held blender in the pan) and blitz until smooth.

Dice the chicken into small cubes, about 1–1.5cm (½–⅝in). Heat 1 teaspoon of the oil in a frying pan (skillet) and when hot add the chicken. Cook for 5–6 minutes on a high heat and then add half of the coriander (cilantro) and season with salt and cracked black pepper.

Cook the onion, peppers and chilli in a hot frying pan (skillet) with the remaining oil for 2–3 minutes. Then, gently reheat the tomato sauce and preheat the grill (broiler) to medium.

Put the tortillas under the grill (broiler) for 20 seconds on each side and immediately transfer to 2 large plates. Spread out a ladle of the sauce onto each tortilla, smooth out to the edges with the back of the ladle.

Next share out the vegetables and chicken between the tortillas and then top with the grated cheese. Put both plates back under the grill (broiler) for 2–3 minutes until the cheese has melted. Garnish with the rest of the chopped coriander (cilantro) and serve straightaway.

Burn Omit the tortilla and turn this filling into a great salad by adding 80g (3¼oz) mixed leaf lettuce or use larger Cos (romaine) leaves to contain the filling within as a salad wrap.

Build Include a side of sweet potato wedges. Preheat the oven to 190°C/375°F/gas mark 5. Wash a small sweet potato and cut into wedges (there's no need to peel). Coat in 1 tsp vegetable oil and a pinch of salt and bake for 20–25 minutes.

Pollo Chayote

By using this South American fruit you bring an interesting dimension to the plate, so serve this dish when the guests are round; it's sure to get them talking. The smoky flavour of the sauce works really well with the sweetness of the peppers and the prickly pear.

Top tip This dish lends itself well to any protein so if chicken's not your thing, try it with fish, tofu or even some crumbled feta.

Sport Packed with a combination of protein and carbohydrate, this makes a great post-exercise dinner.

SERVES 2

80g (scant ½ cup) long-grain brown rice

40g (¼ cup) cooked kidney beans

120g (1 cup) cooked butter (lima) beans (tinned is fine)

80g (3¼oz) edamame (frozen is fine but defrost before use)

2 tsp vegetable oil, for frying

1 small red onion, diced

1 yellow or orange (bell) pepper, diced

2 chicken breasts (a total weight of 280g/10oz)

1 prickly pear

1 tbsp chopped coriander (cilantro)

1 tbsp chopped basil

1 tbsp chopped tarragon

FOR THE SAUCE:

400g (14oz) tin chopped tomatoes

1 clove garlic

½ small onion

1 tsp chipotle paste

¼ tsp ground cumin

½ tsp agave syrup

1 tbsp chopped oregano leaves

First make the sauce. In a pan add all of the ingredients for the sauce apart from the oregano. Bring to the boil then reduce to a simmer and cook for 5 minutes. Remove from the heat and add the oregano. Now, using a hand-held blender blitz the sauce until smooth. Return the pan to a medium heat and reduce the sauce a little more to thicken if necessary. You'll need to reheat to serve, later.

Preheat the oven to 180°C/350°F/gas mark 4. Then, boil several litres (quarts) of water in a large pan and add the rice. Cook for 20–25 minutes until the rice is nearly done. When the rice is almost cooked add both types of beans (kidney and butter/lima beans and edamame) for the final few minutes of cooking. Drain the rice and beans through a sieve (strainer), return to the pan, cover and set aside.

Heat 1 teaspoon of the vegetable oil in a frying pan (skillet) and when hot toss in the onion and peppers. Cook for 2–3 minutes then add these to the pan of rice and beans.

Heat the remaining oil in an ovenproof frying pan (skillet) and when hot cook the chicken breasts until golden brown on one side. Turn them over and pop the frying pan (skillet) into a preheated oven for 10–12 minutes until the chicken is cooked through. Remove from the oven and allow to rest for a few minutes before slicing.

While the chicken is cooking (or even at the start), use a tea (dish) towel to hold the prickly pear (when you buy these the needles on the outer skin will have been removed, but any small ones left can still irritate if you get them in your fingers) and cut into quarters lengthways. Remove the flesh with the knife and dice into small chunks.

Stir the chopped herbs through the rice and bean mixture and divide between 2 plates. Top each pile with the sliced chicken breast, half the sauce and sprinkle over the pieces of prickly pear.

 Burn Leave out the rice and instead serve with a stir-fry of the other ingredients and an extra 40g (1½oz) sliced baby corn and 40g (1½oz) mange tout (snow peas) per portion.

 Build Supersize the amount of kidney beans by 60g (½ cup) per portion.

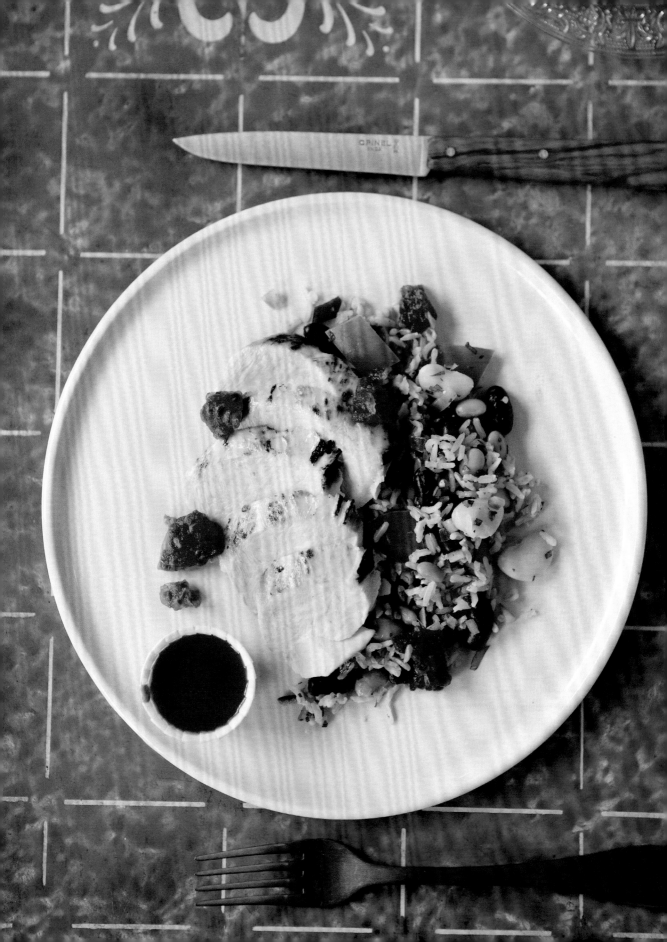

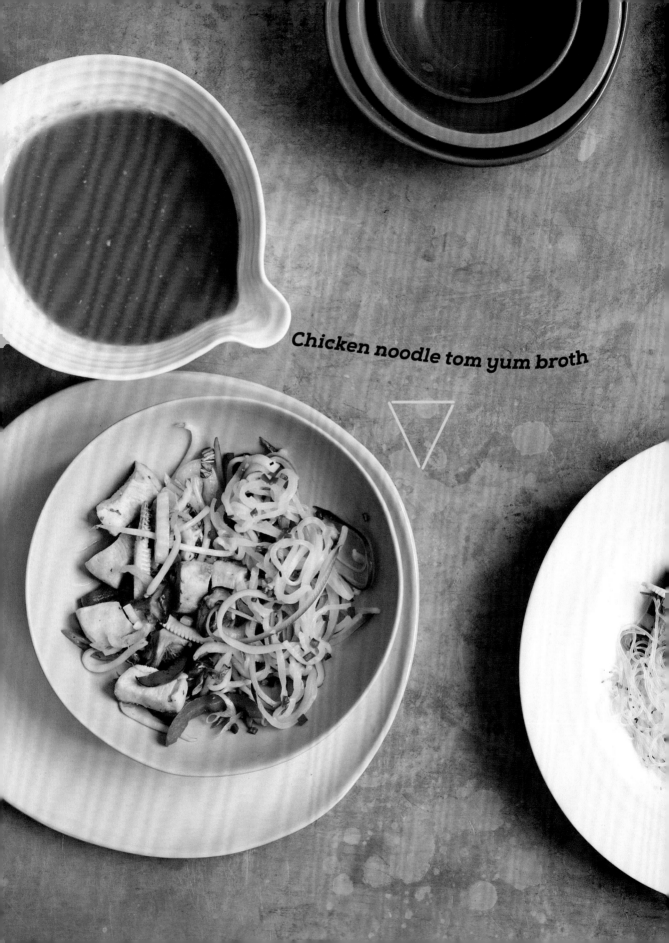

Chicken noodle tom yum broth

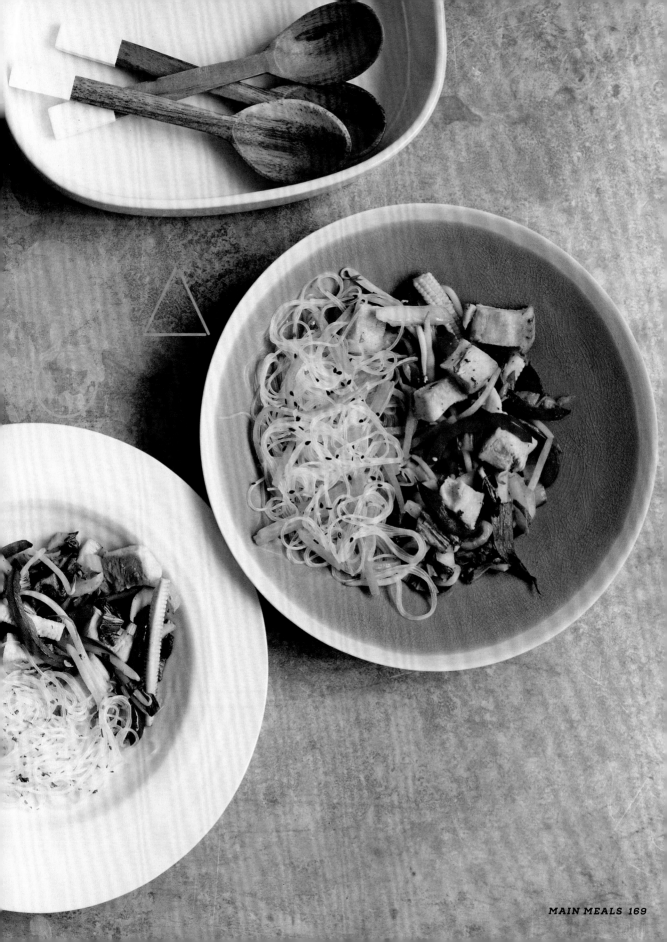

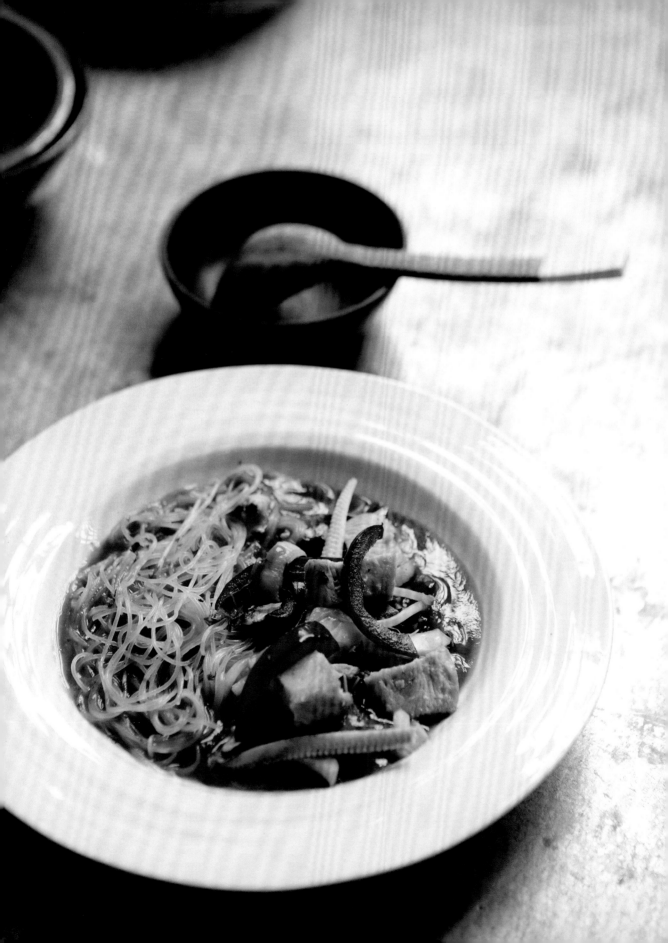

Chicken noodle tom yum broth

An authentic and deliciously nourishing Thai broth. This vegetable-packed dish will help you fight off those nasty bugs in the cold months of the year. Add as much chilli as you wish if you like an extra kick!

Health Stir-frying is one of the best ways to preserve the micronutrient content of vegetables – the quick frying seals in all the goodness.

Top tip Make this dish in the months when colds and flu bugs are doing the rounds, as it's rammed with immunity-supporting ingredients.

SERVES 2

1 pak choi
½ red (bell) pepper
5 baby corn
1 spring onion (scallion)
80g (3¼oz) shiitake mushrooms
20g (scant ¼ cup) coriander (cilantro) leaves
6 mint leaves
100g (3½oz) plum tomatoes
2cm (¾in) piece lemongrass
1 garlic clove
1cm (½in) cube root ginger
½ red chilli
600ml (2½ cups) water
10ml (2 tsp) Thai fish sauce
10g (⅓oz) organic chicken bouillon (1 cube)
2 tsp agave syrup
juice of ½ lime
80g (3¼oz) rice noodles
2 chicken breasts (a total weight of 280g/10oz)
1 tsp vegetable oil
20g (scant ¼ cup) beansprouts

Slice the pak choi, red (bell) pepper, baby corn, spring onion (scallion) and shiitake mushrooms, then finely chop the coriander (cilantro) and mint.

Roughly chop the tomatoes, lemongrass, garlic, ginger and chilli. Put these in a pan along with the water, Thai fish sauce, bouillon, agave syrup, lime juice and half of the coriander (cilantro). Bring to the boil, reduce the heat to a simmer and cook for a further 20 minutes. Using a hand-held blender blitz the contents of the pan until it is as smooth as possible. Set aside.

Cook the rice noodles in plenty of boiling water for 2–3 minutes until soft then drain in a sieve (strainer) and cool under cold running water.

Preheat a large wok over a high heat for 3–4 minutes. Meanwhile, dice the chicken breasts into small cubes. Add the oil to the wok and stir-fry the chicken for 4–5 minutes. Then, add the rest of the sliced vegetables and the beansprouts and cook for a further 2–3 minutes.

Add the 'sauce' from the pan and the noodles and bring back to the boil. Fold in the mint and the rest of the coriander (cilantro) and serve.

▽ **Burn** Replace the rice noodles with courgette 'noodles'. Use a mandolin or a spiraliser to make 80g (3¼oz) courgette (zucchini) 'noodles' per portion. Cook these in a pan of boiling salted water for 2 minutes, drain and serve.

△ **Build** Make some butternut squash 'noodles', using a mandolin or spiraliser, and add these to the rice noodles. Make 80g (3¼oz) squash 'noodles' per portion. Cook in a pan of boiling salted water for 4–5 minutes, until softened, drain and serve.

Feta, turkey and warm lentil salad

The epitome of a classic winter warmer, simple flavours and ingredients come together to create a wholesome, filling and yet moreish dish.

Health Lentils are packed full of fibre and as a result are a great source of low-GI carbs, which is easily forgotten when thinking of healthy carbohydrates.

Sport The dietary nitrates in the beetroots have been shown by research to improve endurance performance. Nothing can stop you now!

SERVES 2

2 carrots

1 large red onion

3 beetroots

1 tsp vegetable oil

½ tsp salt

150g (¾ cup) Puy lentils

250g (9oz) turkey escalope (scallop)

finely grated zest of ½ lemon

10g (⅓oz) chervil, chopped

40g (1½ tbsp) balsamic syrup

100g (3½oz) feta cheese

30g (1oz) baby leaf spinach

Preheat the oven to 180°C/350°F/gas mark 4 and you'll need a baking tray (cookie sheet).

First, prepare the vegetables. Peel the carrots then cut in half lengthways, cut again into pieces on an angle, discarding the tops. Peel and chop the onion into chunky pieces. Peel the beetroot and cut into wedges then cut in half again.

Place all the vegetables on a baking tray (cookie sheet) and toss thoroughly in the oil. Roast in the oven for 50–60 minutes until cooked.

Meanwhile, bring a pan of boiling water to the boil with the measured salt. Pour the lentils into the pan and cook for 18–20 minutes until soft. Then, drain through a sieve (strainer). In a hot, dry ovenproof frying pan (skillet), colour the turkey on one side, turn over and cook in the oven for a further 8–10 minutes. Remove and slice.

Now, bring the salad together by mixing the lentils, carrots, onion, beetroot, lemon zest and two-thirds of the chervil together. Drizzle with the balsamic syrup and add a little salt to taste, if necessary. To serve, divide the spinach leaves between 2 plates and top each with half the lentil-vegetable mixture, half of the turkey slices, feta and remaining chervil and gently toss to combine.

 Burn Replace the lentils with 80g (3¼oz) runner (string) beans per portion that are lightly cooked and thinly sliced. Mix in at the end as you would the lentils.

 Build Add 40g (¼ cup) cooked quinoa per portion and stir through before plating up.

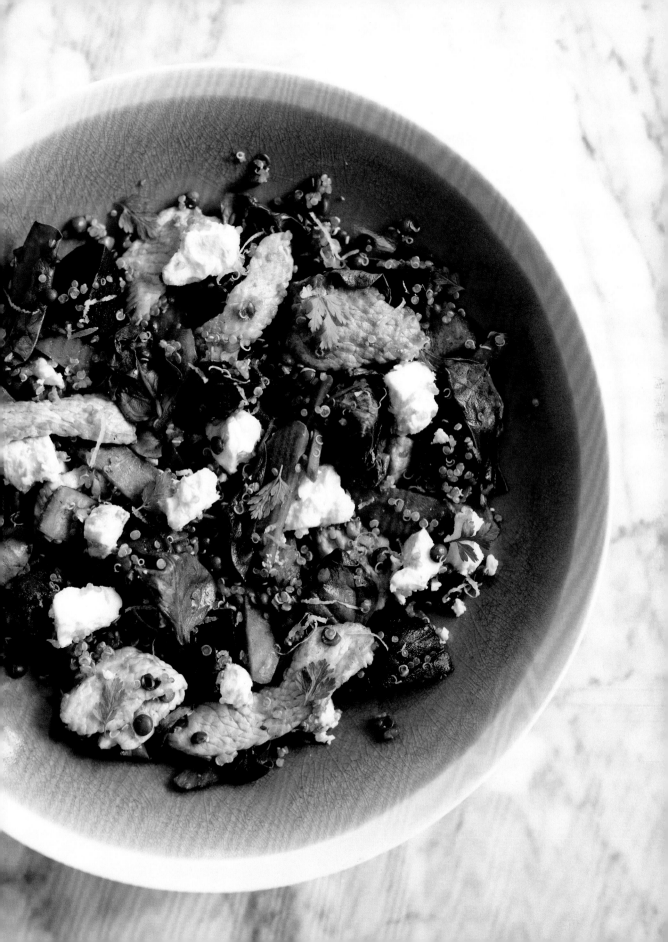

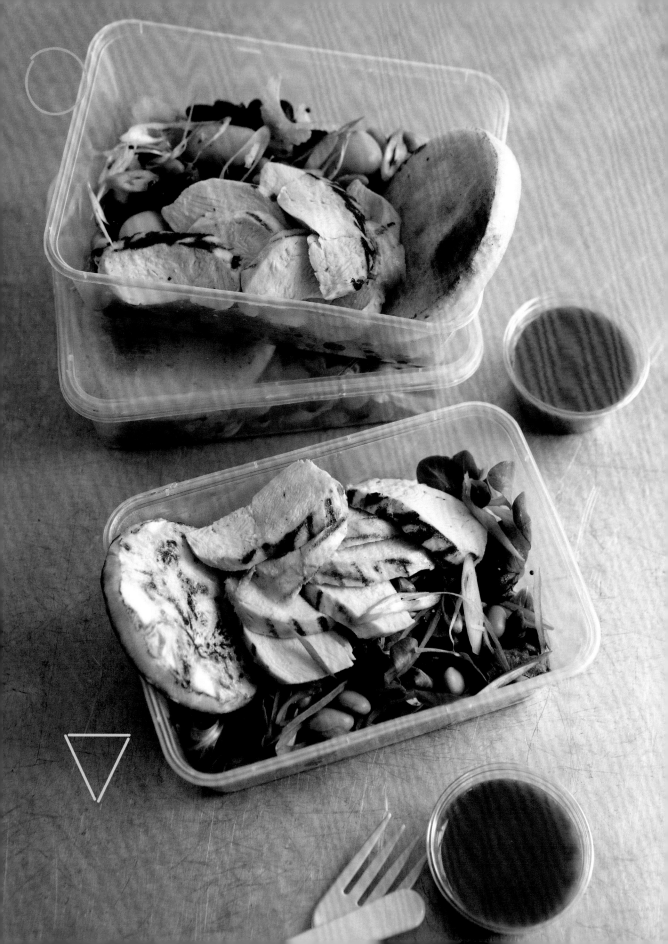

Chicken with roasted yam, bean salad and pepper dressing

Succulent chicken breast with a delicious combo of coconut-roasted yam, a crunchy, fresh bean salad and a knock-out red pepper dressing. Make some for now and pack up the rest for a lunch on the go.

Health Brimming with fibre, potassium and magnesium, yam is a fantastic alternative source of carbs.

Sport The beans are a great source of iron to help support haemoglobin and red blood cell production, creating efficient oxygen transport to the muscles.

SERVES 2

4 yam slices (about 240g/8½oz in total weight)

2 tsp coconut butter

2 chicken breasts (a total weight of 280g/10oz)

¼ stick celery, sliced

1 spring onion (scallion), sliced

60g (scant ½ cup) cooked butter (lima) beans

60g (2¼oz) edamame (frozen ones, defrosted, are fine)

60g (scant ½ cup) cooked black beans

60g (scant ½ cup) cooked kidney beans

FOR THE RED PEPPER DRESSING:

2 red (bell) peppers

1 tsp wholegrain mustard

80ml (⅓ cup) orange juice

½ tsp scotch bonnet pepper sauce, to taste

4 tbsp olive oil

Preheat the oven to 200°C/400°F/gas mark 6, and you'll need 2 baking trays (cookie sheets).

First, make the dressing. Slice the flesh from the peppers discarding the stalk and seeded parts. On a baking tray (cookie sheet) in a preheated oven, roast the peppers for 10–15 minutes until soft. Remove from the oven and allow to cool for 5–10 minutes. Turn the oven down to 170°C/344°F/gas mark 3.

In a blender, add the roasted peppers, wholegrain mustard, orange juice and scotch bonnet pepper sauce and blitz until smooth, then slowly pour in the olive oil. Set aside this dressing.

Peel and trim each slice of yam to about 60g (2¼oz) each. Add these to a pan of salted water and bring to the boil, cook for 5–6 minutes until starting to soften, then drain in a colander.

In a frying pan (skillet) over a medium heat, melt the coconut butter and fry the yam pieces for 2–3 minutes on each side until starting to brown. Transfer to a baking tray (cookie sheet) and roast in a preheated oven for a further 12–15 minutes.

Meanwhile, colour the chicken in the same frying pan (skillet) until golden brown on one side. Transfer the chicken to the baking tray (cookie sheet) in the oven and roast for about 10–12 minutes until cooked (if you have a meat probe the core temperature should be 65°C/149°F).

Mix the celery and the spring onion (scallion) with the beans in a bowl.

To serve, dress the bean salad with some of the red pepper dressing. Slice the chicken and arrange with the yam and salad on 2 plates; pour over a little more dressing, to taste.

Burn Replace the yam with the same weight of celeriac and follow the same method and cooking times. Leave out the butter beans and black beans and, instead, throw in a handful of lamb's lettuce (corn salad) and sliced sugar snap peas per portion to the salad mix.

Build Simply halve the amount of yam used in the recipe.

Parmigiana di melanzane

Oven-baked aubergines (eggplants) packed with rich tomato flavours, nestled with oozing mozzarella and topped with a golden Parmesan crust – what's not to like? It's deliciously moreish yet packed with goodness!

Health This dish provides a well-rounded balance of a large number of vitamins and minerals to keep your body healthy and functioning at its best.

Top tip There's no need to salt aubergines (eggplants) any more to avoid their bitter taste. Modern-day varieties are much less bitter.

SERVES 2

1 aubergine (eggplant), cut into 1cm- (½in-) thick slices
1 courgette (zucchini), cut into 0.5cm- (¼in-) thick slices
½ small onion, chopped
1 tsp roasted garlic paste (see page 106)
400g (14oz) tin chopped tomatoes
1 tbsp chopped oregano
sea salt and freshly ground black pepper
1 slice multi-seeded bread
2 tsp extra virgin olive oil
20g (scant ¼ cup) Parmesan, finely grated
60g (2¼oz) low-fat mozzarella (about ½ a ball)
2 chicken breasts (a total weight of 280g/10oz)
80g (3¼oz) baby plum tomatoes, quartered
2 spring onions (scallions), finely sliced
25g (1oz) baby spinach leaves
25g (1oz) rocket (arugula)
10g (¼ cup) basil leaves, shredded

FOR THE DRESSING:

2 tsp balsamic vinegar
4 tsp extra virgin olive oil

Place the slices of aubergine (eggplant) and courgette (zucchini) into a hot dry frying pan (skillet) and cook until soft and a little charred on both sides (you may need to do this in several batches and keep them warm in the meantime).

Preheat the oven to 180°C/350°F/gas mark 4, and you'll need an ovenproof dish that fits 1.2–1.5 litres (5–6⅓ cups) in and a baking tray (cookie sheet).

Put the onion and roasted garlic paste in a pan with the tomatoes. Bring to the boil and cook until reduced by a quarter and thickened a little. Next, add the oregano and season to taste. Remove from the heat.

In a food processor blitz the bread to a rough crumb then add a teaspoon of the olive oil and mix it in.

In the ovenproof dish spread a little of the tomato sauce on the bottom, then a layer of half of the aubergine (eggplant) and courgette (zucchini) mixture and one-third of the Parmesan. Next, add half of the remaining sauce, the remaining vegetables and top with another third of the Parmesan. Finally, top with the remaining sauce, some slices of mozzarella, the remaining Parmesan and finish with the oiled breadcrumbs. Bake in a preheated oven for 25–35 minutes.

Meanwhile, cook the chicken breasts in a hot frying pan (skillet) with 1 teaspoon of oil until golden on one side, turn the breasts over, transfer to a baking tray (cookie sheet) and bake for 10–12 minutes until cooked (if you have a meat probe the core temperature should be 65°C/149°F). Remove from the oven and slice each into 5 or 6 pieces.

In a large bowl, put the tomatoes, spring onions (scallions), spinach, rocket (arugula) and basil. In a small container with a sealable lid (or jam jar), mix the dressing ingredients together and shake well. Add this dressing to the salad in the bowl and toss until coated.

To serve, place half of the salad onto the side of each plate and top with the pieces of chicken, then divide the parmigiana between the 2 plates.

 Burn Omit the breadcrumb topping and replace with 10g (2 tbsp) chopped pine nuts and 20g (⅛ cup) chopped cooked chickpeas.

 Build For each portion, add an additional sheet of lasagne to each layer or eat with a portion of granary garlic bread.

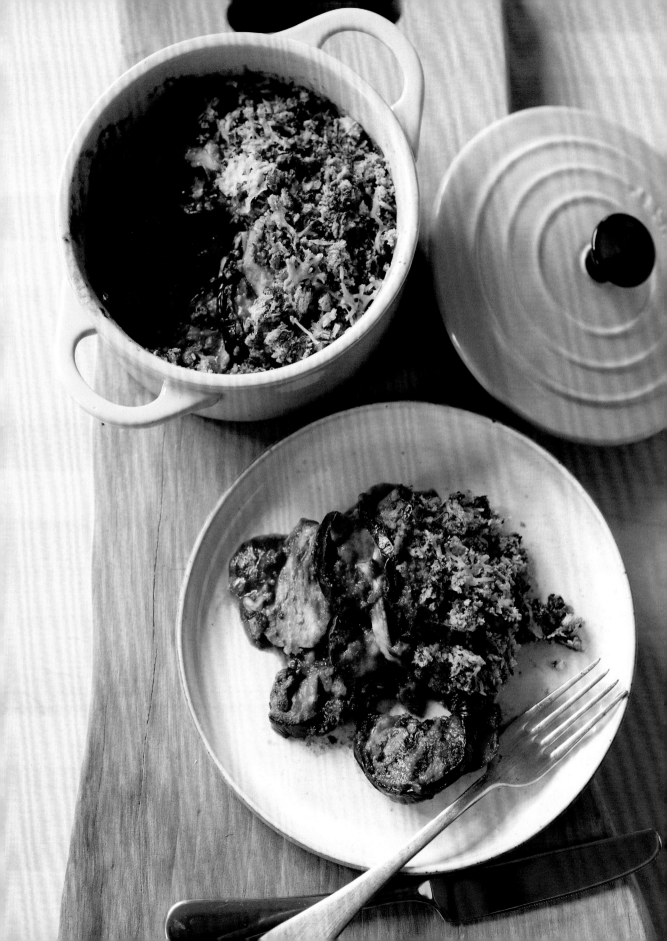

Winter roots korma

This sweet and creamy curry is sure to be a hit with the whole family. Use up whatever vegetables you have lingering around and throw in seasonal ingredients.

Health This curry packs a whole heap of vegetables into one dish – each serving is more than 2 portions of your '5 a day'.

Sport Ginger and turmeric are potent antibiotics and may help reduce infection rate after cuts sustained during sport, especially contact or combat sports.

SERVES 2

½ tsp ground cinnamon

1 tsp ground cumin

1 tsp garam masala

½ tsp ground turmeric

½ tsp ground coriander

1 clove garlic, finely chopped

1.5cm (⅝in) piece root ginger, finely chopped

200ml (scant 1 cup) coconut milk

¼ tsp chilli (red pepper) flakes

5g organic vegetable bouillon (½ cube or 1½ tsp powder)

50g (½ cup) ground almonds

80g (3¼oz) broccoli

80g (3¼oz) cauliflower

80g (3¼oz) celeriac

80g (3¼oz) sweet potato

1 tsp vegetable oil

300g (10½oz) turkey escalope (scallop), cut into thin strips

40g (1½oz) spinach leaves

sliced red chilli, to garnish

In a large frying pan (skillet), dry toast the spices over a medium heat for 3–4 minutes.

Next, add the garlic, ginger, coconut milk, chilli (red pepper) flakes, bouillon and the ground almonds to the pan. Bring to the boil and reduce the heat to a simmer and cook for 5–6 minutes.

Break the broccoli and cauliflower into small florets, and peel and dice the celeriac and sweet potato.

Cook the celeriac and sweet potato in a large pan of boiling water for 4 minutes. Then, add the cauliflower and broccoli and cook for a further 4 minutes. Drain in a colander.

Preheat a large frying pan (skillet) over a high heat with the oil and cook the turkey strips for 3–4 minutes. Next, add the cooked vegetables and cook for 3 minutes. Then, add the spinach along with the coconut milk 'sauce', continue to cook until the spinach has wilted.

Divide the korma between 2 bowls, garnish with sliced red chillies and serve straightaway.

 Burn Replace the sweet potato with a 50g (⅓ cup) portion of small diced carrot. Add these at the beginning of cooking, along with the ginger and garlic.

 Build Give yourself a portion of rice (60g/⅓ cup uncooked weight) per person or enjoy a chapatti as well.

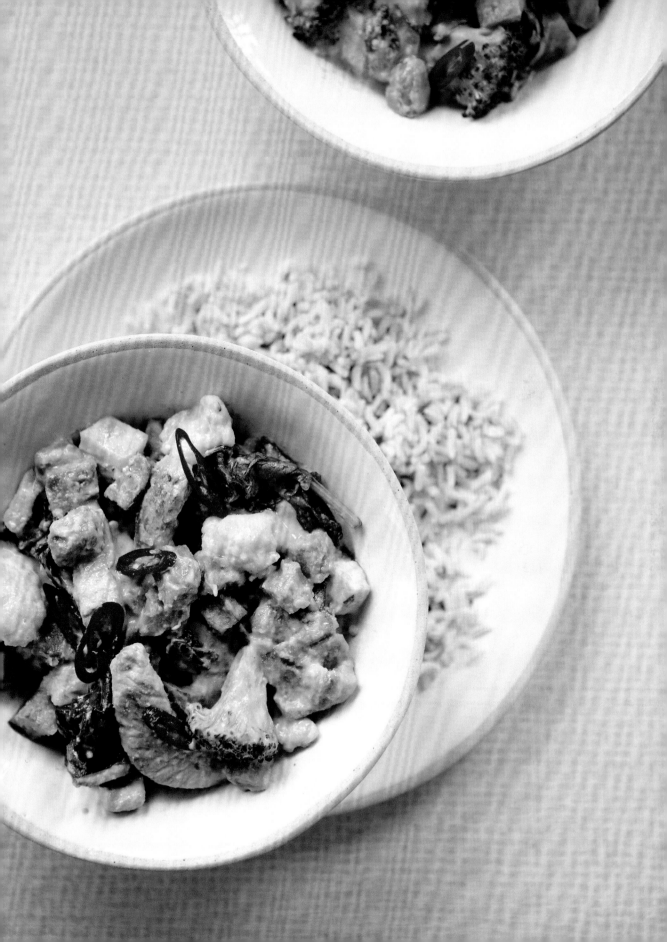

▽ **Burn** Follow the recipe (see opposite), but omit the quinoa and instead add 500g (1lb 2oz) lamb's lettuce (corn salad). There's no need to mix the purée in with the replacement lettuce, so just use it as a dressing for the salad as a whole.

△ **Build** Follow the recipe (see opposite), but add 50g (⅓ cup) cashew nuts and 30g (¼ cup) cooked chickpeas or 30g (¼ cup) toasted pine nuts, whichever you prefer.

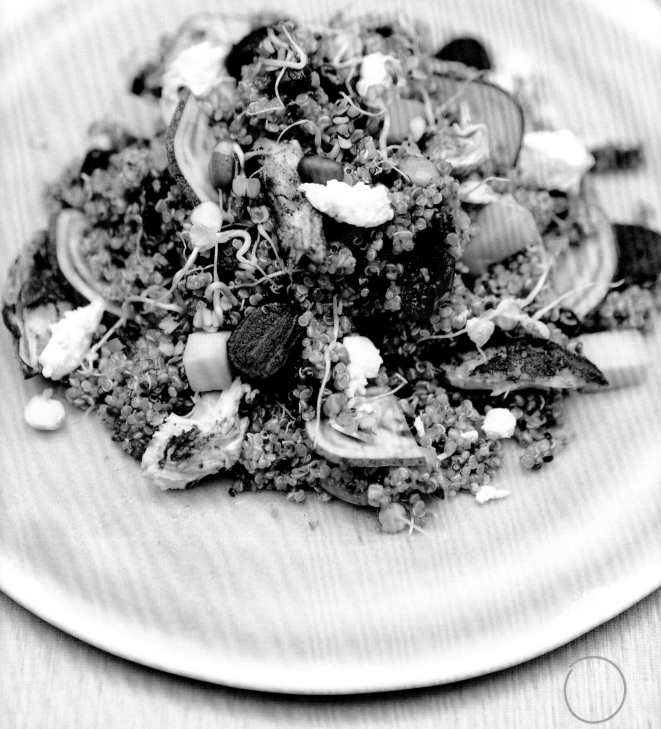

Super-green candy salad with mango and pomegranate

You almost feel healthier simply by looking at this plate of fresh food, but do eat it because it's delicious and oh-so good for you. If you don't eat meat, then try this dish with tofu pieces instead of the chicken.

Health The phenolic compounds found naturally in mangoes can help protect against certain forms of cancer.

Sport Quinoa is a very slow-release form of carbohydrate, perfect for fuelling training sessions.

SERVES 2

FOR THE 'SAUCE':

60g (2¼oz) baby leaf spinach

10g (⅓oz) mint

10g (⅓oz) coriander (cilantro)

20g (¾oz) spring onion (scallion)

¼ red chilli

25ml (1½ tbsp) extra virgin olive oil

FOR THE SALAD:

200g (generous 1 cup) raw quinoa (400g/2¼ cups in cooked weight)

140g (5oz) chicken breast

salt and black pepper, to season

extra virgin olive oil, for oiling

50g (1¾oz) edamame

20g (¾oz) Peppadew peppers, quartered

100g (3½oz) mango, peeled and cut into chunks

45g (1½oz) pomegranate seeds

45g (1½oz) candy beetroot, peeled and finely sliced

45g (1½oz) golden beetroot, peeled and finely sliced

45g (1½oz) feta cheese

rose sprouts or alfalfa sprouts, to garnish

First, make the 'sauce'. Place everything into a blender and blitz to make a purée and set aside. This sauce will be used later to transform the colour of the cooked quinoa into a gorgeous and vibrant green.

Cook the quinoa in boiling water for 15 minutes. When cooked, drain and leave it to cool down.

Slice the chicken breast along its length so you get a butterflied joint. Season, lightly oil and cook in a frying pan (skillet) over a medium heat for 4 minutes on each side. Remove from the heat and shred the chicken.

Now, in a large bowl, mix the 'sauce' you made earlier with the cooked quinoa. Then toss in all the prepared fruits and vegetables together, mix and, lastly, crumble in the feta. To serve, divide between 2 plates, top with the shredded chicken and garnish with rose sprouts.

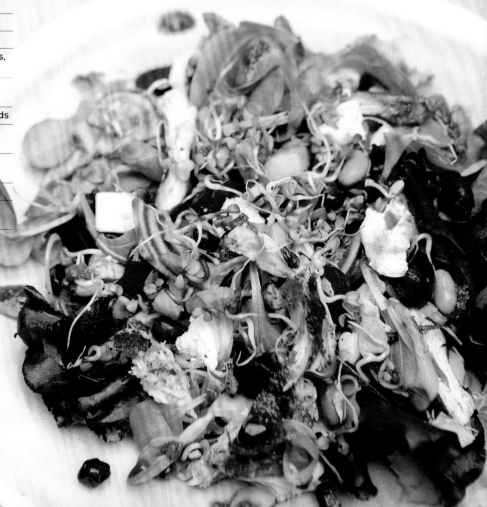

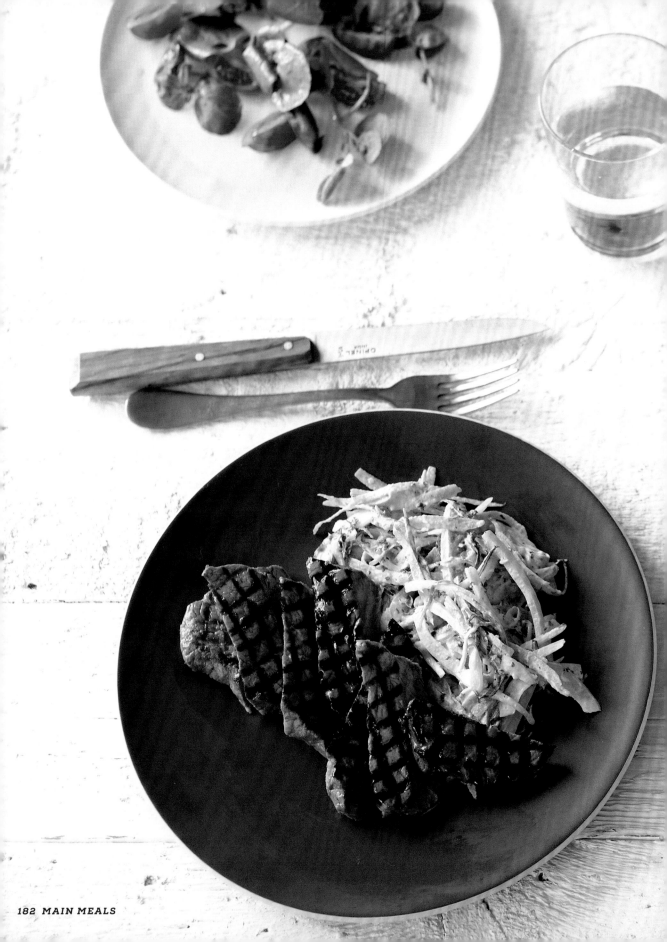

Steak and salsify chips with chicory slaw

Our take on the classic steak and chips! If you can't get hold of salsify then parsnips work just as well. Serve any leftover coleslaw with lunch the next day; keep in an airtight container until you're ready to eat.

Health Salsify is a relatively low-carb root vegetable, which helps prevent any spiking of blood sugar after this meal.

Sport The iron in the steak can help keep red blood cells working at full potential, thereby providing an efficient source of oxygen to working muscles.

SERVES 2

2 sirloin steak (200g/7oz each), trimmed of excess fat

1 tsp olive oil, for brushing

2 tsp honey

¼ tsp Dijon mustard

120g (4½oz) baby plum tomatoes, halved

30g (1oz) watercress

¼ tsp freshly ground black pepper

80ml (⅓ cup) olive oil

juice of ½ lemon

FOR THE SLAW (MAKES ENOUGH FOR 4):

1 carrot

10g (⅓oz) fresh horseradish

1 head white chicory, sliced lengthways

1 head red chicory, sliced lengthways

¼ onion, sliced

120g (½ cup) crème fraîche

1 tsp white wine vinegar

2.5g (¾ tbsp) chopped parsley

FOR THE CHIPS:

400g (14oz) salsify, peeled and cut into chips

40g (⅓ cup) polenta

¼ tsp salt

Preheat the oven to 180°C/350°F/gas mark 4, and you'll need 2 baking trays (cookie sheets).

First, make the slaw, grate the carrot and the horseradish into a bowl and add the chicory and the onion. Mix in the crème fraîche, white wine vinegar and chopped parsley; keep the 2 extra portions (this slaw serves 4) in an airtight container in the fridge, where it'll keep for 3 days.

Put the salsify chips in a pan of cold water, bring to the boil and cook until they start to soften. Drain in a sieve (strainer) and roll in a mixture of the polenta and salt. Transfer to the baking tray (cookie sheet) and bake in a preheated oven for 12–15 minutes until starting to colour.

Preheat a heavy-bottomed frying pan (skillet) or griddle over a high heat for 5 minutes. Brush the steaks with a little of the oil. Cook in the frying pan (skillet) for a few minutes on each side until the desired colour is achieved. Transfer to a baking tray (cookie sheet), pop in the oven and cook until done to your liking.

Meanwhile, in a beaker mix the honey and Dijon mustard together.

Remove the steaks from the oven and, using a pastry brush, glaze with a little of the honey and mustard mixture and set aside to rest.

In a bowl, put the tomatoes with the watercress. Using a hand-held blender, blitz the black pepper, oil and lemon juice into the honey and mustard mix, use a little of this to dress the tomato and watercress salad.

To serve, use one-quarter (not half) of the slaw per portion and arrange on a plate with half of the salad, chips and the steak.

▽ **Burn** Replace the salsify chips with the same weight of celeriac chips, cooked in the same way but no need to boil them first.

△ **Build** Serve with a side of steamed whole corn on the cob.

Beef and vegetable tagine with cauliflower 'couscous'

Here is one of my all-time favourite one-pot wonders! The slow-cooked beef falls apart and the sweetness of the apricot and pomegranate complements it so well. A real hearty dish, perfect on a cold winter's evening!

Health Cauliflower is a good source of choline, which may boost cognitive function and diminish the decline in memory that often comes with age.

Sport Why not use the cauliflower 'couscous' in other dishes as an innovative and tasty swap for higher-carb couscous.

SERVES 2

FOR THE BRAISED BEEF TAGINE:

2 tsp vegetable oil

300g (10½oz) beef chuck, diced

½ tsp ground cinnamon

½ tsp ground allspice

¼ tsp ground ginger

¼ tsp ground cumin

¼ tsp paprika

400g (14oz) tin chopped tomatoes

1 tbsp tomato purée (paste)

5g organic chicken bouillon (½ cube)

250ml (generous 1 cup) water

80g (3¼oz) butternut squash, cut into 1cm (½in) cubes

½ pomegranate

½ onion, chopped

1 clove garlic, chopped

30g (scant ¼ cup) dried apricots, sliced

50g (⅓ cup) cooked chickpeas

sea salt, to taste

FOR THE CAULIFLOWER 'COUSCOUS':

220g (7½oz) cauliflower (about 1 small cauliflower)

1 tsp chopped coriander (cilantro)

finely grated zest of ½ lemon

Add 1 teaspoon of oil to a very hot frying pan (skillet) followed by the beef and cook for 3–4 minutes until browned all over. Add the spices and cook for a further 2–3 minutes, then transfer into the ceramic bowl of a slow cooker, and then add the tomatoes, tomato purée (paste), bouillon and the water. Put the lid on and cook on the low setting for 8–10 hours until very tender. (If you don't have a slow cooker, use an ovenproof dish with a lid and cook in the oven (at a low temperature, about 90°C/194°F/gas mark ¼) for the same length of time.)

Drain the beef and any remaining tomato pieces (nearly all of this will have broken down) into a sieve (strainer) over a bowl. Keep both the beef mix in the sieve (strainer) and the cooking liquor and set aside.

Meanwhile, cook the butternut squash in a pan of boiling water until tender, drain and set aside.

Hold the pomegranate over a bowl firmly and tap the back of it with a rolling pin (or wooden spoon) until all the seeds fall out.

Add 1 teaspoon of oil to a hot frying pan (skillet) over a high heat and toss in the onions and cook until browned. Then, add the garlic, apricots, chickpeas and the cooking liquor from the beef. Reduce this to the consistency of a sauce and season with salt to taste. Finally, add the beef and tomato mixture and the squash and heat through.

Next, make the 'couscous'. Break the cauliflower into florets, put into the bowl of a food processor and pulse until it has broken into small pieces the size of the grains of couscous. Tip out onto a tray and pick any larger pieces out. Add to a large pan of boiling water and cook for 2½ minutes. Drain and mix in the coriander (cilantro) and the lemon zest.

To serve, divide the 'couscous' between 2 plates or bowls, top with the beef tagine and garnish with the pomegranate seeds.

Burn Swap out the butternut squash and the chickpeas from the recipe and replace with 40g (⅓ cup) diced carrot and 40g (⅓ cup) diced courgette (zucchini). Cook the carrots in a pan of boiling water until tender and dry fry the courgette (zucchini) for 3–4 minutes. Add these to the sauce before serving.

Build Replace the cauliflower with 80g (scant ½ cup) couscous (uncooked weight) per portion.

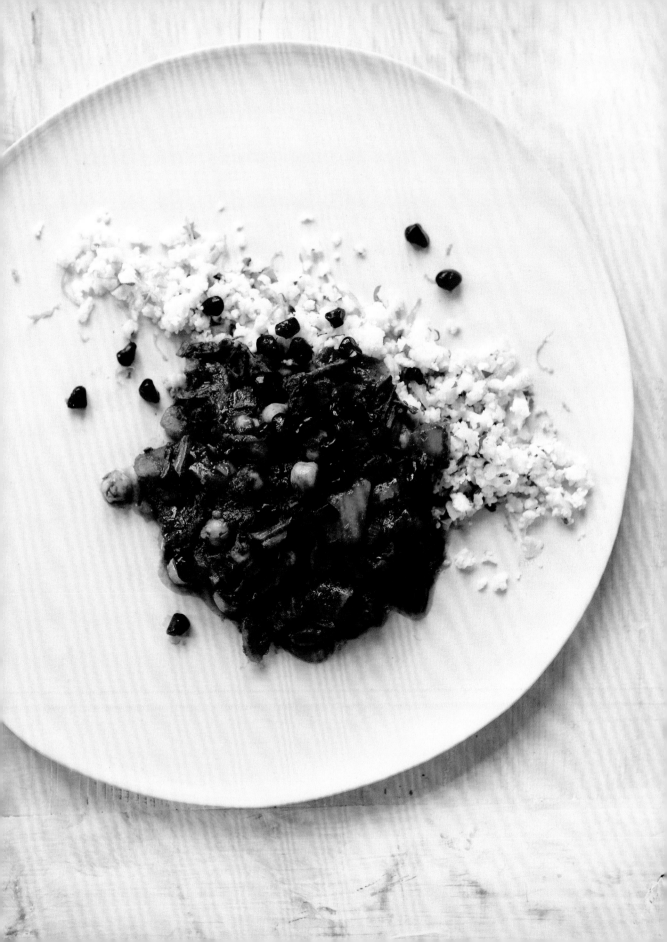

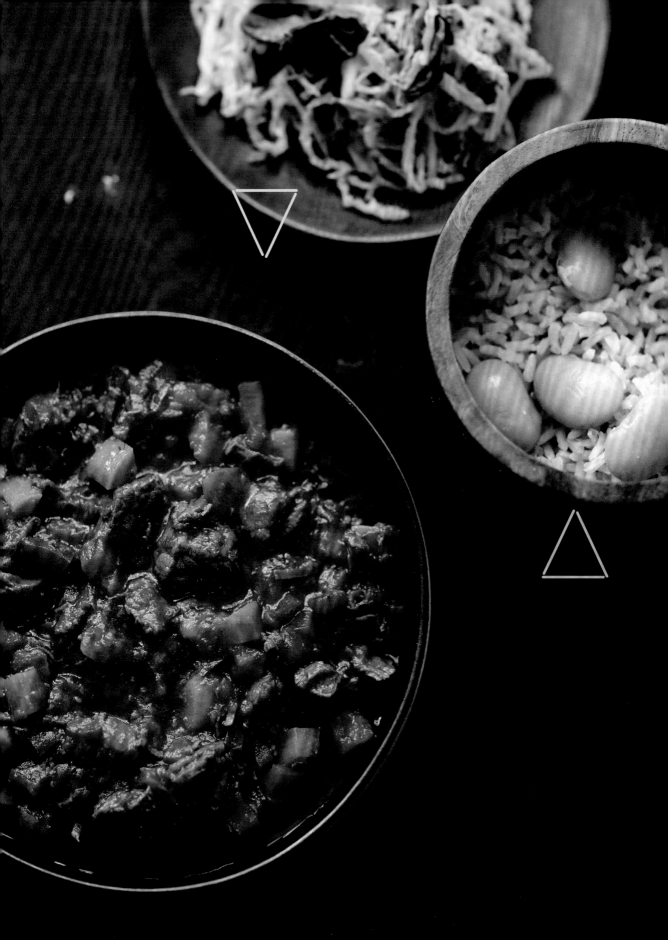

Hungarian beef goulash and rice

This dish is brimming with flavour. It may seem like a long cooking time but once the beef is in the slow cooker (or low oven), you can just leave it to work its magic.

SERVES 2

- 2 tsp vegetable oil
- 250g (9oz) beef chuck, diced
- 400g (14oz) tin chopped tomatoes
- 1 tbsp tomato purée (paste)
- 200ml (scant 1 cup) water
- 15g (½oz) organic beef bouillon (1½ cubes)
- 1 onion
- 2 small red (bell) peppers
- 60g (2¼oz) carrot
- 2 tsp paprika
- chilli (red pepper) flakes (optional), to taste
- 30g (scant ¼ cup) plain (all-purpose) flour, sifted
- 80g (⅓ cup) short-grain brown rice
- salt and cracked black pepper
- 1½ tsp roasted garlic paste (see page 106)
- 60g (¼ cup) natural yogurt, plus extra to garnish
- 1 sprig of flat-leaf parsley, chopped, to garnish

Into a very hot frying pan (skillet) add 1 teaspoon of the oil along with the beef for 3–4 minutes until browned all over. Transfer into the ceramic bowl of a slow cooker, and then add the tomatoes, tomato purée (paste), water and bouillon. Put the lid on and cook on the low setting for 8–10 hours until very tender. (If you don't have a slow cooker, use an ovenproof dish with a lid and cook in the oven (at about 90°C/194°F/gas mark ¼) for the same length of time.)

Strain the beef and any remaining tomato pieces (nearly all of this will have broken down) into a sieve (strainer) over a bowl. You'll end up with some cooking liquor and pieces of beef.

Dice the onion, peppers and carrots. In a large, hot frying pan (skillet) pour in the remaining oil, add the roasted garlic paste and the vegetables, spices and flour. After 1 minute, turn down to a medium heat and cook for a further 3 minutes. Slowly pour in the beef liquor, stirring continuously, then add the beef. Allow to simmer until the sauce has reduced to a coating consistency.

While the sauce is thickening, cook the rice. Bring a large pan of water to the boil with a little salt, to taste, add the rice and reduce the heat when the water has come back to the boil. Cook for 22–25 minutes, making sure that the rice is well covered in water. When cooked, drain.

When the sauce has thickened, remove it from the heat and pour all of the yogurt into one side of the frying pan (skillet), stir the yogurt into the sauce gradually. Add a little salt and cracked black pepper, to taste.

To serve, divide the rice and the goulash in half and arrange on 2 plates, then garnish with a little extra yogurt and the parsley.

 Burn Replace the cooked rice with 80g (½ cup) steamed, shredded Savoy cabbage and steamed 40g (1½oz) spinach per portion.

 Build Heat through 80g (½ cup) cooked butter (lima) beans per portion and add to the rice.

Braised lamb fattoush

Celebrate summer all-year with this Lebanese salad – its tangy taste comes from the vibrant red sumac and the lemon. And it's a great way of using up slightly stale pitta breads.

Health Sumac is most commonly found in its powdered form but is processed from berries. It has a host of health benefits, being antifungal, antimicrobial, antioxidant and anti-inflammatory.

Top tip The yellow pointed pepper is the traditional pepper used in this salad but if you can't get hold of one of those, simply use a yellow bell pepper instead.

SERVES 2

1 tsp vegetable oil

500g (1lb 2oz) boned leg of lamb joint

½ stick celery, roughly chopped

¼ onion, roughly chopped

1 small carrot, roughly chopped

½ tsp sumac

¼ tsp ground cumin

2 tsp roasted garlic paste (see page 106)

5g (⅛oz) organic chicken bouillon (½ cube)

750ml (3⅓ cups) water

2 wholewheat pitta breads

sea salt and freshly ground black pepper

1 pointed yellow pepper, diced

⅓ cucumber, diced

140g (5oz) cherry tomatoes, halved

½ banana shallot (Echalion), finely sliced

1 baby gem (Boston) lettuce, finely sliced

2 tsp mint leaves, chopped

finely grated zest and juice of ¼ lemon

2 tsp extra virgin olive oil

80g (½ cup) cooked chickpeas

Preheat a large, heavy-bottomed pan over a high heat for 5 minutes. Preheat the oven to 120°C/250°F/gas mark ½.

Put the vegetable oil and the lamb into the pan to colour the joint on all sides. Add the chopped vegetables and continue to cook for a further 4–5 minutes. Next, add the sumac, cumin, garlic paste, bouillon and water to the pan. Transfer the contents into a lidded casserole dish and cook in the oven for 6 hours.

Meanwhile, cut the pitta into squares of about 1.5cm (⅝in), place on a baking tray (cookie sheet) and bake in the oven for 60–80 minutes until completely dried out. Remove from the oven and set aside.

When the lamb is ready, drain the meat and vegetables in a sieve (strainer) over a bowl, add 5–6 ice cubes to the bowl of cooking liquor then discard the vegetables and let the meat cool for 5–10 minutes. When the ice has melted, use a spoon to skim off the fat that has risen to the surface. Pour the liquor into a pan and reduce to 75ml (5 tbsp).

Use a fork to shred the meat on the leg of lamb into medium-sized pieces, removing any remaining fat as you do so. Add the reduced liquor to the meat and season to taste.

In a large bowl, mix the pepper, cucumber, tomatoes, shallot, lettuce, mint and lemon zest together and dress with the lemon juice and olive oil. Then, fold in the chickpeas and pitta pieces. To serve, divide the salad between 2 bowls and top with the lamb.

Burn Follow the recipe above but don't include the pitta bread.

Build Allow an extra half a pitta bread per portion when making the pitta pieces.

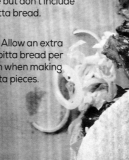

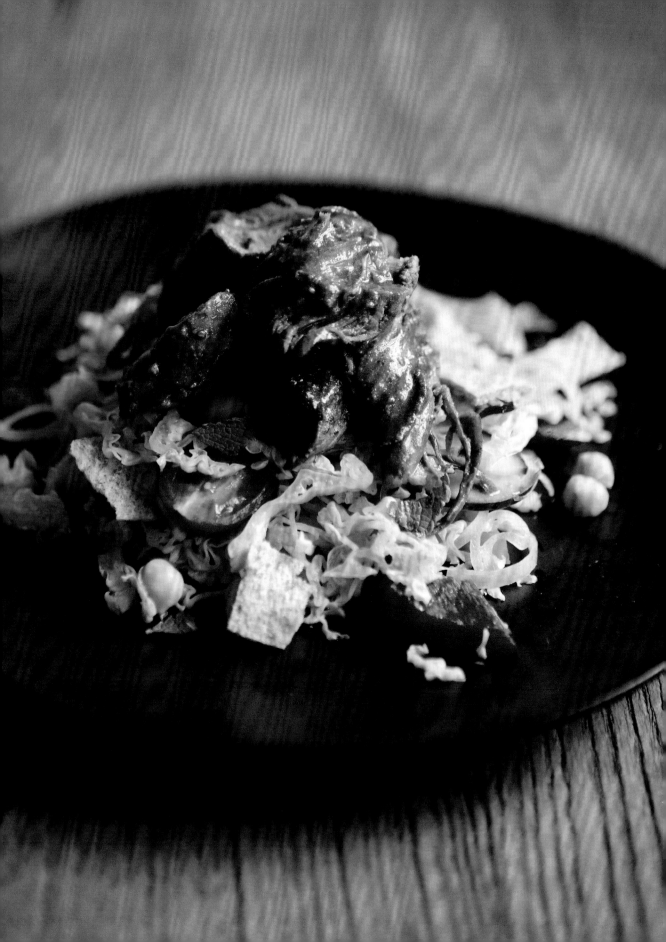

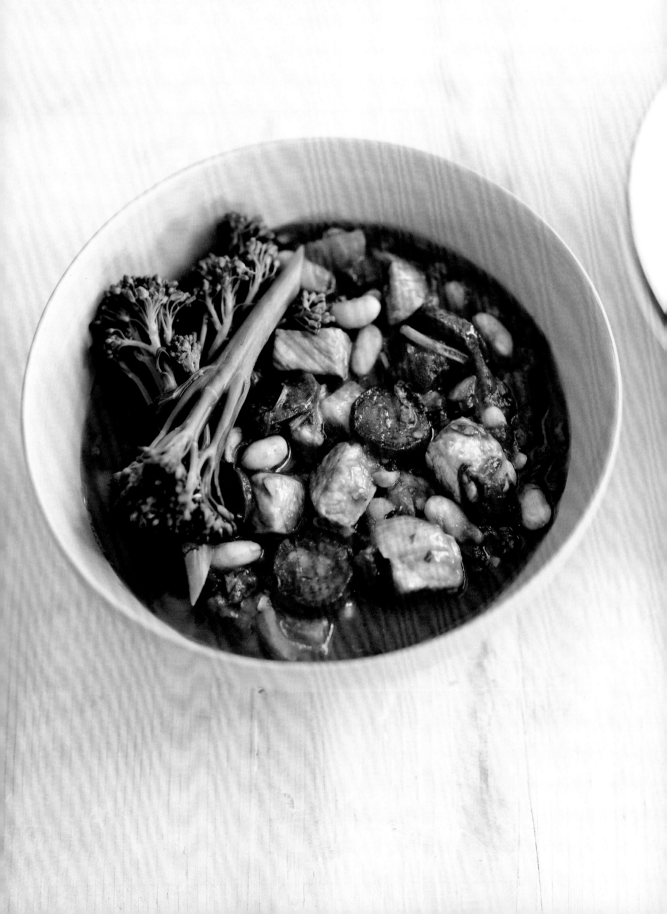

Pork cassoulet

Try this wonderfully flavoursome and filling pork dish with gutsy chorizo, beans and tomatoes. It's easy to make and ideal for the whole family.

Health Pork is a great source of selenium, which is required for correct reproduction and thyroid function, as well as being an antioxidant.

Top tip If you are not a meat eater, replace the pork with more beans. You will still have a high-protein meal, which is now even lower in fat!

SERVES 2

1 tsp extra virgin olive oil
50g (1¾oz) chorizo, diced
½ onion, diced
220g (7½oz) pork fillet (tenderloin), cut into 1cm (½in) cubes
1 clove garlic, finely chopped
400g (14oz) tin chopped tomatoes
220g (1½ cups) cooked cannellini beans
1 tbsp tomato purée (paste)
5g organic vegetable bouillon (½ cube or 1½ tsp powder)
1 tsp agave syrup
½ tsp cornflour (cornstarch)
50ml (scant ¼ cup) water
20g (¾oz) spinach leaves
1 sprig parsley
1 tsp thyme leaves, picked
160g (5½oz) tenderstem broccoli

Preheat a large pan over a high heat, add the oil, chorizo, onion and pork and cook for 3–4 minutes. Next, add the garlic, tomatoes, beans, tomato purée (paste), bouillon and agave syrup to the pan.

In a cup, mix the cornflour (cornstarch) with the water and add to the pan. Stirring well, bring to the boil then reduce the heat to a simmer and continue to cook for 10–12 minutes.

Chop the spinach and add this with the parsley and the thyme for the last 2–3 minutes of cooking.

Cook the broccoli in a pan of boiling water over a high heat for 3 minutes. Drain and serve immediately.

To serve, divide the cassoulet between 2 bowls and serve the tenderstem broccoli alongside.

 Burn Remove the beans and replace with 100g (¾ cup) diced parsnip per portion. Add to the pan when you would add the beans.

 Build For each serving, include 80g (3¼oz) sweet potato, cut into 1cm (½in) cubes, added to the pan at the beginning with the pork.

Skinny sausage stew with root vegetables and dumplings

Enjoy this comforting one-pot stew that's delicious and healthy – perfect for sharing at the dinner table.

Health This dish is packed with selenium from the pork and semolina. Not many dumplings are good for you, but these are!

Top tip Select handmade sausages from trusted butchers (not the cheaper products in supermarkets) for high-quality lean sausages.

SERVES 2

½ onion, chopped

1 carrot, diced

¼ celeriac (about 140g/5oz), diced

1 parsnip, diced

1 tsp vegetable oil

a pinch of salt

4 low-fat pork sausages or 8 low-fat pork chipolatas

15g (1 tbsp) butter

10g plain (all-purpose) flour

250ml (1 cup) water

400g (14oz) tin chopped tomatoes

10g (⅓oz) organic chicken bouillon (1 cube)

1 tsp roasted garlic paste (see page 106)

1 tsp Worcestershire sauce

4 sage leaves

1 tsp chopped tarragon

FOR THE DUMPLINGS:

1 egg, separated

50g (¼ cup) semolina

20g (¼ cup) buckwheat flour

¼ tsp salt

a pinch of black pepper

1 tsp chopped rosemary

2 tsp olive oil

Preheat the oven to 220°C/425°F/gas mark 7, and you'll need 2 baking trays (cookie sheets).

Toss the onion and root vegetables in the oil and salt and tip into a baking tray (cookie sheet). Roast in a preheated oven for 20–25 minutes until they have a good amount of colour. Remove and set aside.

Place the sausages onto a baking tray (cookie sheet) and cook in the oven until golden brown. Remove and set aside.

In a large ovenproof pan, melt the butter over a low heat, add the flour then return to the heat and cook for 3–4 minutes. Remove from the heat and slowly mix the water in a little at a time. Next, add the tomatoes, bouillon, garlic, Worcestershire sauce and herbs. Bring to the boil and add the roasted vegetables and sausages. Put into the oven and turn the temperature down to 180°C/350°F/gas mark 4. Cook while you get on to make the dumplings.

Meanwhile, in a bowl, mix the egg yolk with the semolina, buckwheat flour, salt, pepper, rosemary and olive oil. In a separate bowl, whisk the egg white to soft peaks and gently fold the whites into the rest of the ingredients until mixed well.

Remove the pan from the oven. Divide the dumpling mixture into 4 and, using 2 spoons together, shape each dumpling into a quenelle and sit them on top of the stew. Return the pan to the oven and cook for 15–18 minutes until the dumplings are golden.

To serve, divide the stew between 2 bowls, giving each half of the sausages and half of the dumplings.

 Burn Remove the dumplings and serve with 60g (2¼oz) broccoli per portion.

 Build Serve with 150g (5½oz) portion of steamed new potatoes, tossed with some chopped chives, a little roasted garlic paste and a drizzle of extra virgin olive oil. Season, to taste.

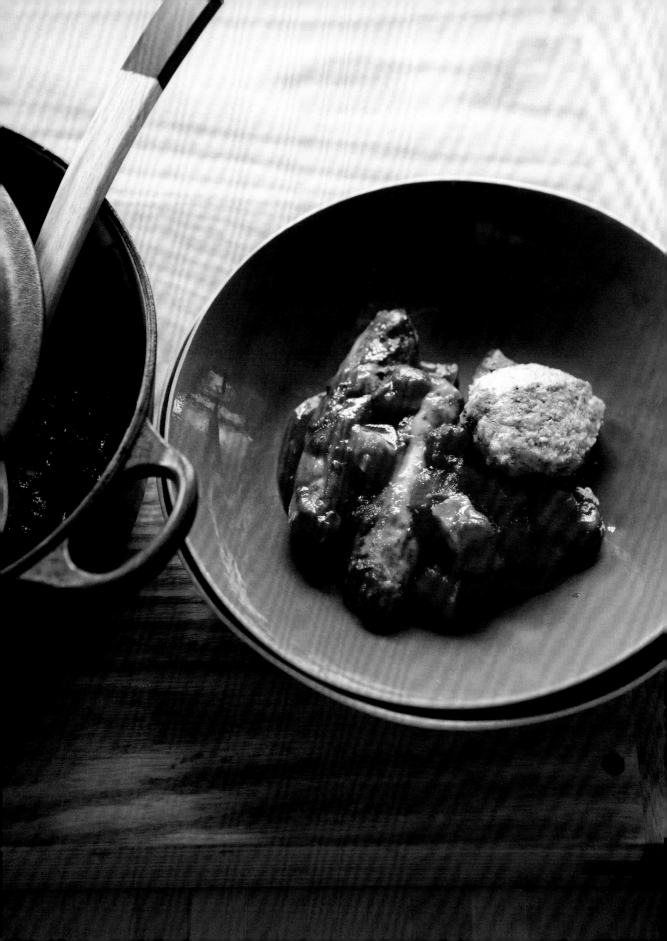

Creole gumbo with red beans and rice

This Louisiana-inspired classic is a staple of the Deep South in the US, but this version has a few Soulmatefood tweaks so is much better for you.

Health The dish is crammed with fibre thanks to the brown rice and kidney beans – it's a superb meal to support gut function and digestion.

Sport A great recovery meal that can be made before a session and heated through after for a quick and effective meal after exercise.

SERVES 2

80g (scant ½ cup) long-grain brown rice

100g (⅔ cup) cooked kidney beans (tinned is fine)

2 spring onions (scallions), finely sliced

600ml (2½ cups) water

12g (⅓oz) organic chicken bouillon (1¼ cube)

2 tsp vegetable oil, plus 1 tsp for frying

40g (¼ cup) plain (all-purpose) flour

100g (3½oz) saucisson, skin removed and diced

1 onion, diced

2 green (bell) peppers, sliced

2 sticks celery, sliced

3 cloves garlic, chopped

2 tsp Cajun seasoning

½ tsp smoked paprika

10 raw king prawns (shrimp), shelled

½ tsp Tabasco sauce or hot pepper sauce

½ tsp Worcestershire sauce

Boil several litres (quarts) of water in a large pan and add the rice. Cook for 20–25 minutes until the rice is nearly done. Then, add the beans for the final few minutes of cooking. Drain the rice and beans through a sieve (strainer) and return to the pan along with the spring onions (scallions) and stir to mix. Cover and set aside until the sauce is done.

Meanwhile, bring half of the measured water to the boil in a pan then stir in the bouillon and the rest of the water. Turn off the heat.

Heat 2 teaspoons of vegetable oil in a large pan over a medium heat. Add the plain (all-purpose) flour and stir it into the oil using a wooden spoon until it forms a paste. Continue cooking, stirring all the time, until it turns a golden brown colour. Remove from the heat and add a small amount of the stock, stir in until well combined; repeat adding a little stock at a time until all the liquid is combined (a blitz with a hand-held blender in the pan will banish any lumps).

Heat 1 teaspoon of vegetable oil in a deep frying pan (skillet) on a high heat. Fry the vegetables for 2–3 minutes, then add the dry spices and stir for another minute.

Next, add the prawns (shrimp) and pour on the stock. Then add the Tabasco and Worcestershire sauces and bring to the boil. Simmer for 3–4 minutes and then divide between 2 plates.

 Burn Remove the rice portion and make a warm salad. Use spring onions (scallions) along with 30g (1oz) spinach leaves and 40g (1½oz) green beans, blanched and sliced. Season with salt and dress with lemon juice and cracked black pepper.

 Build To the rice, add an extra 40g (¼ cup) kidney beans and 80g (3¼oz) roasted diced sweet potato per portion.

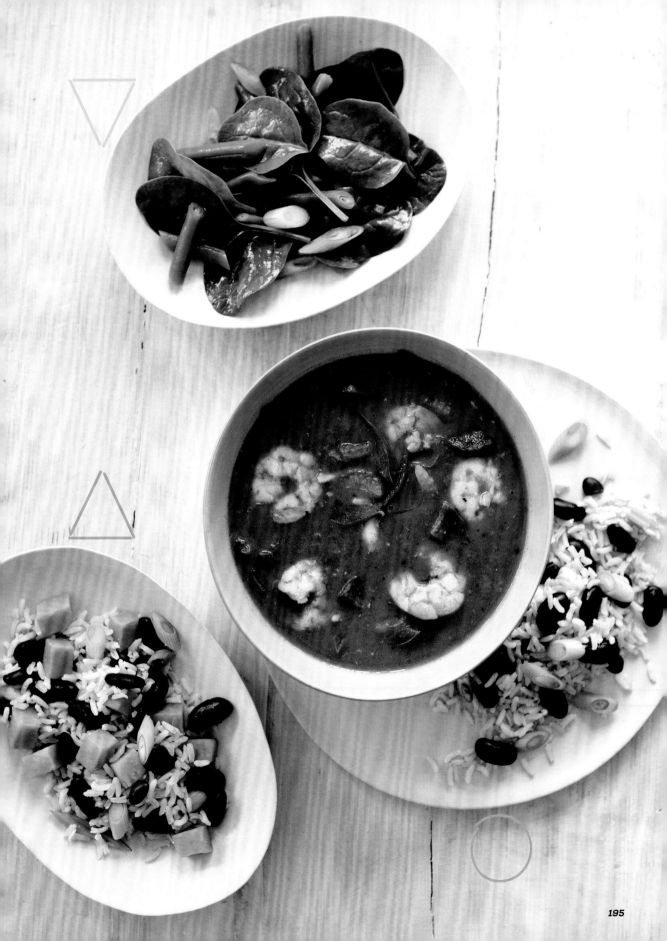

Ham-wrapped cod with pickled cherries, kale and potato

Serve up this sophisticated dish for a romantic meal or dinner party. The intense saltiness of prosciutto works so well with the cod. And all topped off, well bottomed off actually, on a bed of baked potato and apple.

Health In general the darker a fruit, the higher its antioxidant potential. Choosing black cherries increases the antioxidant content of this dish.

Sport One fillet of cod can provide more than your daily requirement of selenium – an antioxidant that can help protect against training stress.

SERVES 2

400g (14oz) small potatoes (Estima or Vivaldi)

1 Granny Smith apple

sea salt, to taste

2 cod fillets (about 160g/5½oz each)

2 slices prosciutto

60g (2¼oz) kale, leaves removed from the stems

1 tsp butter

½ tsp roasted garlic paste (see page 106)

FOR THE MARINADE:

100ml (scant ½ cup) cider vinegar

70g (scant ¼ cup) honey

15 juniper berries

10 black cherries, pitted and halved

FOR THE SAUCE:

120g (½ cup) crème fraîche

1½ tsp honey

1 tsp Dijon mustard

1 tsp cider vinegar

2 tsp chopped dill

40ml (1½ tbsp) whole milk

First, make the marinade. In a beaker with a hand-held blender, blitz the cider vinegar with the honey, then add the juniper berries and blitz very quickly to break up the berries a little. Add the cherries and leave to infuse for at least 4 hours.

Preheat the oven to 160°C/325°F/gas mark 2½, and line a 450g (1lb) loaf tin as well as a lidded ovenproof dish (it needs to be big enough to fit the fish in) with baking parchment.

Peel the potatoes and the apple and thinly slice using a mandolin. In the prepared loaf tin, layer half the potato slices, then the apple slices and top with the rest of the potato; season with a little salt between each layer. Place a piece of baking parchment on top of the potato and bake in a preheated oven for 45–50 minutes until done. Remove from the oven and allow to cool in the tin.

Meanwhile, wrap each piece of cod in a slice of prosciutto and place in the prepared ovenproof dish. Pop it in the oven, alongside the potato and apple bake, for 15–18 minutes until done.

Cook the kale in a pan of boiling water for 4–5 minutes until softened. Drain through a sieve (strainer) and squeeze out any excess water with the back of a spoon. Melt the butter in the pan, add the roasted garlic paste and the kale then mix well and season with salt, to taste.

In another pan make the sauce. Bring the crème fraîche, honey, Dijon mustard, vinegar, dill and milk quickly to the boil, stirring, and serve.

To serve, cut the potato and apple bake in half and arrange one half on each plate. Sit a piece of cod on top, scatter half of the cherries on each plate, divide the kale and pour the sauce over the cod.

Burn Replace the potatoes with celeriac and reduce the cooking time by 10 minutes.

Build Increase the portion size of the potato stack by increasing the ingredients by 50 per cent per portion.

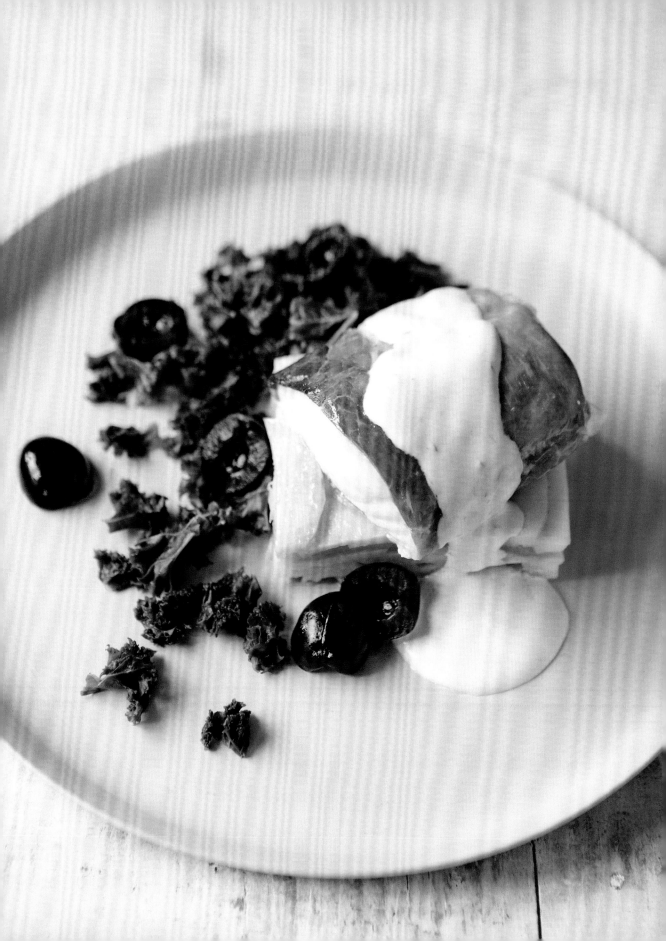

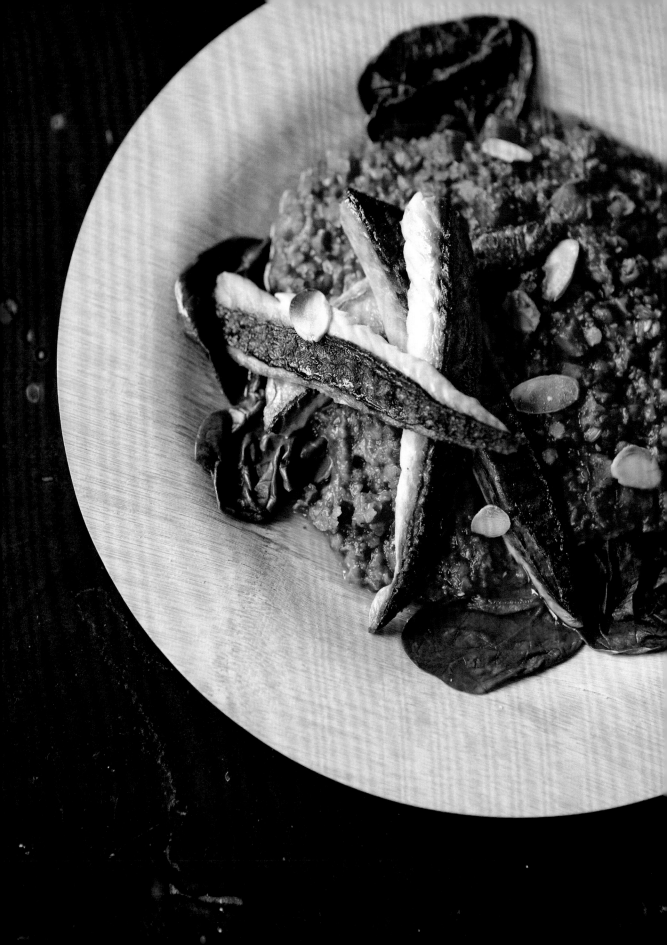

Mackerel masoor dahl

Inexpensive, healthy and super-tasty, this masoor dahl is the perfect comforting dinner. This wholesome dish is quick and easy to make and its warming spices will certainly keep the cold away!

Health The Indian spices and ingredients provide great antibacterial properties and make a super dish to help maintain your body's immunity.

Sport Mackerel is an excellent source of omega-3 fatty acids, helping reduce both inflammation and the chance of injury during training and competing.

SERVES 2

½ small onion, diced
1 large carrot, diced
2 tsp vegetable oil
100g (½ cup) red lentils
400g (14oz) tin chopped tomatoes
1 tbsp tomato purée (paste)
1 tsp chopped root ginger
2 cloves garlic, chopped
1½ tsp garam masala
1 tsp fennel seeds
½ tsp ground turmeric
¼ tsp chilli (red pepper) flakes
10g (⅓oz) organic vegetable bouillon (1 cube or 3 tsp powder)
400ml (1¾ cups) water
2 mackerel fillets (a total of 200g/7oz in weight)
60g (2¼oz) spinach leaves
juice of ½ lime
6g (⅛oz) coriander (cilantro) leaves, chopped
20g (scant ¼ cup) almonds, toasted, to garnish

Cook the onion and carrot in a large pan with 1 teaspoon of the oil over a medium heat for 4–5 minutes until the onion is soft.

Add the lentils, followed by the tomatoes, tomato purée (paste), all the spices, bouillon and water. Bring to the boil and then simmer. Cook until the lentils soften and break down to thicken the sauce – about 25–30 minutes. The sauce should be quite thick when it's done.

Cut the mackerel fillets lengthways down the middle and trim away any small bones and the dark blood line. In a hot non-stick frying pan (skillet) over a medium heat with the remaining oil, lay the fillets skin side down and cook for 3–4 minutes, then turn over and cook for a further minute.

Meanwhile, in a frying pan (skillet) wilt the spinach over a medium heat for 30–40 seconds.

To serve, stir the lime juice and chopped coriander (cilantro) into the cooked dahl and divide between 2 bowls, top with half of the mackerel and spinach and then sprinkle over the toasted almonds.

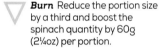

Burn Reduce the portion size by a third and boost the spinach quantity by 60g (2¼oz) per portion.

Build As this dish is based around lentils, which are quite high in carbohydrates, you can just increase the portion size to 60g (⅓ cup) uncooked rice or add a chapatti to the meal.

Causa santa rosa core ingredients

For Balance, replace the quinoa with some cubed, cooked butternut squash and new potatoes.

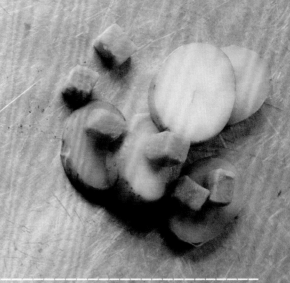

For Build, follow the recipe using quinoa and cubes of sweet potato.

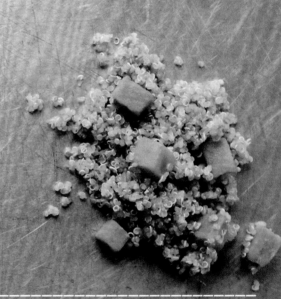

For Burn, replace the quinoa with dressed little gem (Boston) leaves and diced mango.

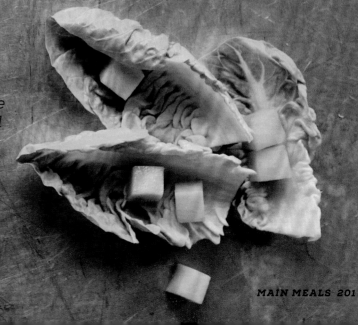

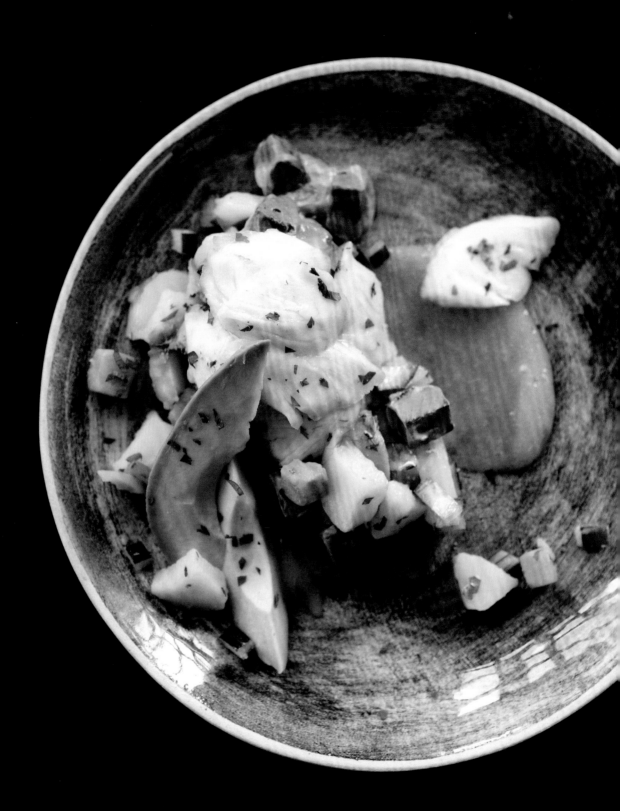

Causa santa rosa

Traditionally, causa santa rosa is a layered potato dish from Peru. Here we've given it the Soulmatefood treatment and partnered it with some fragrant and tangy ceviche – another specialty of Peru.

Health Limes pack a powerful punch of vitamin C and, what's more, contain powerful flavonoid compounds that have been shown to be antibiotic and may even combat cancer.

Sport Quinoa is a high-protein grain with a high nutritive value, making this a perfect post-training session dish to help your body recover and be in peak fitness the next day.

SERVES 2

80g (½ cup) quinoa
220ml (scant 1 cup) water
a pinch of salt
1 small sweet potato, peeled and diced
¼ red onion, finely diced
2 tsp chopped coriander (cilantro), plus extra to garnish
2 tsp chopped mint
1 cooked beetroot, diced
3 tbsp crème fraîche
½ tsp crushed pink peppercorns
sea salt, to taste
1 ripe avocado
flesh of 1 small mango

FOR THE CEVICHE:

1cm (½in) cube root ginger
2 cloves garlic
½ red chilli
10g coriander (cilantro) (a small bunch)
juice of 1 lemon, plus extra for avocado
juice of 4 limes
2 sea bass fillets, skinless and boneless (100g/3½oz each)

Burn Replace the quinoa with little gem (Boston) leaves and diced mango pieces and toss these with a dressing made from chopped mint and coriander (cilantro), lemon juice and olive oil.

Balance Replace the quinoa with chilled, cooked butternut squash and new potatoes that have been diced. Use 100g (3½oz) of each per portion and toss this with a dressing made from chopped mint and coriander (cilantro), lemon juice and olive oil.

First, make the ceviche liquor. Roughly chop the ginger, garlic, chilli and coriander (cilantro) then place in a small container with the lemon and lime juice. Place a lid on the container and give it a good shake. Leave in the fridge to infuse for 30 minutes. Strain through a fine sieve (strainer) sitting atop a bowl and place in the fridge.

Put the quinoa into a sieve (strainer) and rinse under cold water, then transfer into a pan with a lid and add the water and salt. Bring to the boil then reduce the heat to a simmer. Cook until all the water has been absorbed and the quinoa is light and fluffy. Add a little more boiling water, if necessary. When done transfer to a flat baking tray (cookie sheet) and allow to cool for 10 minutes before chilling.

Cook the sweet potato in a small pan of boiling water until soft but not falling apart. When done drain and run under cold water until chilled.

Put the red onion in a bowl along with the quinoa, sweet potato and the chopped herbs. Mix together and set aside.

Then, mix the beetroot cubes with the crème fraîche, pink peppercorns and a little salt, to taste.

Halve the avocado and remove the stone. Cut each half into quarters lengthways and use a knife to remove the skin. To avoid any browning, squeeze a little lemon juice over each piece.

Place the mango pieces into a beaker and using a hand-held blender blitz until you have a smooth purée.

Now, using the sharpest knife you have (don't use a serrated one), slice the fish fillets in half lengthways and cut away the dark-coloured blood line. Slice the fish into (about 1cm/½in) pieces along the grain of the fish.

Remove the bowl and sieve from the fridge and discard the contents of the sieve. Place the pieces of fish into the citrus juice mix, making sure each is fully covered by the liquor and leave to cure for 10 minutes. Then, remove the fish pieces from the liquor and serve.

To assemble, onto each plate put 1 dessertspoon of mango purée and spread across the plate a little, using the back of the spoon. Next to this, pile half of the quinoa mix (you can do this in a ring if you want it neat). Now put the beetroot mix on top and the avocado to the side of this. Place the ceviche on top and garnish with chopped coriander (cilantro).

Sea bass with roasted vegetables and butter bean sauce

This fragrant summer meal is light but packed with flavour. The samphire complements the sea bass perfectly and the butter beans add a delightful creamy texture to the dish.

Health Sea bass provides a good hit of phosphorus, which is crucial for DNA and RNA and energy production and transport in the body.

Top tip If you prefer a more rustic dish then lightly mash the butter beans, rather than puréeing them to give more texture.

SERVES 2

1 tsp roasted garlic paste (see page 106)

2.5g organic vegetable bouillon (¼ cube or ¾ tsp powder)

100g (⅔ cup) cooked butter (lima) beans

200ml (scant 1 cup) water

3 tsp extra virgin olive oil

150g (5½oz) butternut squash, cut into 4cm x 1cm x 1cm (1½in x ½in x ½in) batons

1 red (bell) pepper, sliced

1 small red onion, sliced

1 tsp chopped thyme

sea salt

2 sea bass fillets (about 150g/5½oz each)

2 heads pak choi, cut in half lengthways

2 tsp chopped flat-leaf parsley

juice of ¼ lemon

40g (1½oz) samphire

Preheat the oven to 200°C/400°F/gas mark 6, and you'll need a baking tray (cookie sheet).

In a small pan, heat the roasted garlic paste, bouillon and butter (lima) beans with the water and bring to the boil. Transfer to a blender and blitz until you get a smooth sauce; slowly add 1 teaspoon of the oil and a little more water, if necessary. Return to the pan and cover with a lid.

Toss the squash in 1 teaspoon of the oil and place on a baking tray (cookie sheet). Bake in a preheated oven for 20 minutes. After that time, add the pepper, onion, thyme and a pinch of salt and toss again. Return to the oven and cook for a further 10 minutes.

In a preheated non-stick frying pan (skillet) over a medium–high heat, add the last of the olive oil and gently place the sea bass fillets skin side down. (When putting the fillets into the pan gently press them down using a spatula for a few seconds, this will keep the fish flat and help it cook evenly.) Turn the heat down to medium and cook for 3–4 minutes on this side.

Meanwhile, cook the pak choi in a large pan of boiling water. Cook for 2–2½ minutes then drain and dry on kitchen paper (paper towels).

Gently return the bean sauce to the boil and add the chopped parsley and salt, to taste.

Now, turn the fish over and place the pak choi in the pan cut-side down and cook for a further 2 minutes. Squeeze the lemon juice over the fish and add a pinch of salt, to taste. Blanch the samphire in boiling water for 30 seconds and drain. To serve, divide all of the vegetables between the 2 plates, drizzle over the sauce, top with the fish and finally garnish with the samphire.

Burn Replace the squash with the same weight of lightly cooked carrot batons. Cook as for the squash.

Build Add an 80g (3¼oz) portion of sweet potato batons per portion. Cook these the same as for the butternut squash.

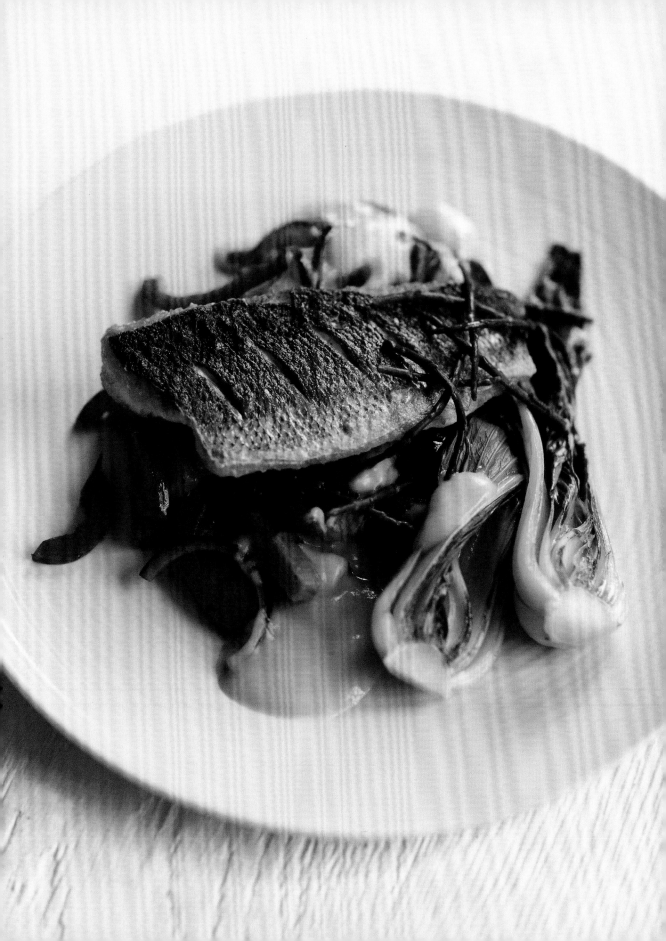

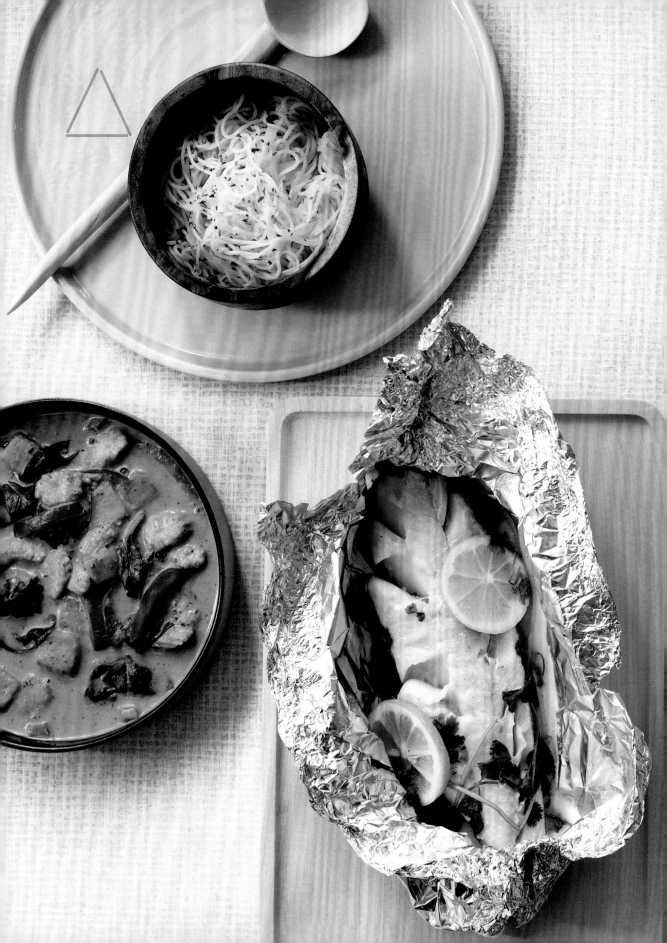

Thai red fish curry

Thai food can be one of the healthiest ways to cook vegetables; this fragrant authentic dish will have your taste buds tingling while giving your body all the nutrients that it needs.

Health Coconut milk is a great source of medium chain triglycerides (known as MCTs), which can help boost cognitive brain functions.

Top tip If you're having friends or family over, prepare the veg and fish parcels in advance. Then you only have to heat the sauce and place the fish in the oven.

SERVES 2

FOR THE THAI RED CURRY PASTE (MAKES ABOUT 200G OF PASTE):

4 medium red chillies

2 tsp cumin seeds

4 tsp coriander seeds

2 tsp grated fresh ginger

1 star anise

6 whole cloves

4 stems lemongrass, trimmed and chopped

4 shallots

6 cloves garlic

finely grated zest and juice of 2 limes

2 tsp hot paprika

FOR THE CURRY:

200ml (scant 1 cup) tinned coconut milk

200g (7oz) tin chopped tomatoes

1 tbsp tomato purée (paste)

1 tsp fish sauce

1 tsp tamari (or soy sauce)

5g organic vegetable bouillon (½ cube or 1½ tsp powder)

juice of ½ lime

1 sweet potato

2 tsp vegetable oil

1 small red (bell) pepper

60g (2¼oz) sugar snap peas

80g (3¼oz) baby corn

2 fillets haddock or other white fish (total weight 240g/8½oz)

25g (½ cup) coriander (cilantro) leaves and stalks, separately chopped

2 slices of lemon

½ tsp coriander seeds

sea salt flakes

50g (1¾oz) baby spinach leaves

30g (¼cup) cashew nuts

Deseed and chop the chillies. Toast the cumin and coriander seeds in a frying pan (skillet) and blitz in a food processor or spice mill until a fine powder. Add the rest of the curry paste ingredients and blitz to a smooth paste. Put this paste into an airtight container and store in the fridge.

For the curry itself, put the coconut milk, chopped tomatoes and tomato purée (paste) into a blender and blitz for 3 minutes. Strain through a fine sieve (strainer) into a pan; push it through, if necessary, with the back of a spatula.

Add the fish sauce, tamari and vegetable bouillon and bring to the boil. Add 1 heaped teaspoon of the red curry paste and the lime juice, and stir in well then taste; add more as necessary.

Preheat the oven to 180°C/350°F/gas mark 4. Meanwhile, peel and dice the sweet potato, place on a baking tray (cookie sheet) and coat with 1 teaspoon of the oil. Bake in a preheated oven for 20–25 minutes until cooked and golden. Then turn the oven temperature up to 200°C/400°F/gas mark 6.

Thinly slice the pepper, sugar snap peas and the baby corn. Cook in a hot frying pan (skillet) with the remaining oil for 2–3 minutes.

Wrap the fish fillets, coriander (cilantro) stalks, lemon slices and coriander seeds inside a domed foil parcel (it should look like a huge silver Cornish pasty). Bake the parcel in a preheated oven for 10–12 minutes. Remove from the oven and open the parcel then, sprinkle a little sea salt over each fillet. To serve, line the bottom of 2 large bowls with the spinach leaves and divide the vegetables between the 2 and pour over the sauce. Pull the fish fillets apart into large chunks and arrange on top, garnish with the chopped coriander (cilantro) leaves and cashew nuts.

▽ **Burn** Replace the sweet potato with 80g (3¼oz) roasted diced aubergine (eggplant).

 Build Supersize by adding 40g (1½oz) rice noodles per portion. Add the noodles to a pan of boiling water and cook for 2½–3 minutes until soft. Drain and serve.

Goat's cheese risotto with smoked salmon and beetroot

This risotto is full of flavour and very satisfying; it makes a great mid-week dinner. If you're not a fan of goat's cheese, swap it for any low-fat soft cheese.

Health Vitamin B12 in the salmon is vital for energy metabolism and brain function. This meal provides plenty of B12, keeping you alert and full of energy.

Sport This dish provides a great combination of omega-3s, calcium and dietary nitrates to give a well-rounded nutrient profile to help improve endurance.

SERVES 2

- 200ml (scant 1 cup) beetroot juice
- 40g (1½oz) cooked beetroot, diced
- ½ celeriac (about 300g/10½oz in weight), peeled
- 5g organic vegetable bouillon (½ cube or 1½ tsp powder)
- 500ml (2 cups) boiling water
- ¼ onion, finely chopped
- 1 clove garlic, finely chopped
- 2 tsp extra virgin olive oil
- 120g (½ cup) arborio risotto rice
- small sprig of rosemary, chopped
- 2 tbsp crème fraîche
- 80g (⅓ cup) soft goat's cheese
- sea salt, to taste
- 50g (1¾oz) baby spinach leaves
- 150g (5½oz) cold-smoked salmon

In a small pan over a medium heat, reduce the beetroot juice to about one-eighth of its volume (just under 2 tablespoons), then stir in the diced beetroot. Remove from the heat and set aside.

Slice the celeriac on a mandolin using the julienne attachment, then chop into small dice. Cook in a pan of boiling water for 3–4 minutes until just starting to soften. Drain through a sieve (strainer) and set aside.

Dissolve the bouillon in a jug (pitcher) with the boiling water.

Heat the onion and the garlic along with the olive oil in a large pan and gently cook over a low heat for 5–6 minutes until the onion is soft. Add the rice and turn the heat up to medium-high. Stir this for 1 minute until the rice is coated in the oil and starts to look transparent on the outside. Add 100ml (scant ½ cup) of the stock and continue to stir, making sure the rice does not stick to the pan. Once the liquid has been absorbed, add another 100ml (scant ½ cup) and repeat until the stock is used or the rice is cooked (about 20 minutes). The rice should still have a firm texture in the centre; if you run out of stock before the rice is ready use boiling water instead.

When the rice is cooked, add the celeriac, chopped rosemary and crème fraîche then crumble in the goat's cheese and add salt to taste. Next, gently fold in the beetroot.

Wilt the baby spinach leaves in a large pan with a lid over a high heat; this will only take 30–40 seconds.

To serve, pile half of the spinach onto each plate along with half of the risotto and top with the smoked salmon.

 Burn Double up on the celeriac per portion to replace the rice.

 Build Replace the celeriac with a double portion of rice.

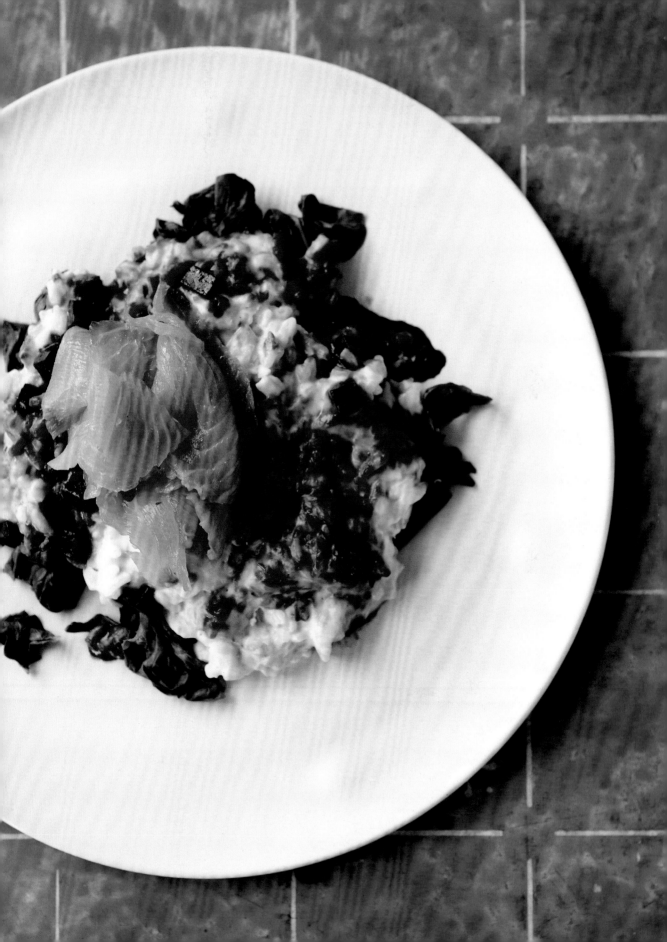

Smoked salmon with goat's cheese salad and mead dressing

This salad is a real winner when you want to impress guests! The balance of colours and textures looks great on the plate and the salmon and goat's cheese are balanced by the clean taste of fennel and cucumber.

Health The salmon is rich in DHA, which can help maintain and even improve brain health and reduce the risk of degenerative brain diseases.

Top tip Use the same salad base and top with other lean proteins, such as prosciutto or cooked chicken breast.

SERVES 2

- 180ml (scant 1 cup) mead (if you can't source mead, use 170ml/¾ cup white wine with 10g/2 tsp honey)
- 2 rye crackers (such as Ryvita)
- 40g (scant ¼ cup) soft goat's cheese
- 60g (¼ cup) low-fat cream cheese
- 16 asparagus tips
- ½ fennel bulb (about 150g/5½oz)
- ¼ cucumber
- 6 radishes
- ¼ stick celery
- 2 spring onions (scallions)
- 2 cooked beetroots
- 2 tsp chopped chervil or sweet cicely, plus extra to garnish
- 2 tbsp cold-pressed rapeseed (canola) oil
- 2 hot-smoked salmon fillets (about 240g/8½oz in total)

In a small pan bring the mead (or wine and honey) to the boil and reduce to about 2 tablespoons worth in volume.

Meanwhile, in a beaker crush the rye crackers with the end of a rolling pin to form a rough crumb texture and tip into a small bowl.

Mix the cheeses together in a bowl with a wooden spoon. Using two teaspoons, scoop a little of the mix onto one and use the other to push the mix into a quenelle. Drop this into the cracker crumbs and roll around until well coated, remove and set aside. Repeat until all the mixture is used (you want an even number of these quenelles – 6 or 8).

Cook the asparagus in a pan of boiling water for 3 minutes, then drain in a sieve (strainer) and plunge into a bowl of iced water until cold. Drain in the sieve (strainer).

Using a mandolin, finely slice the fennel, cucumber, radish and celery. Using a knife finely slice the spring onions (scallions) and beetroot. Set the beetroot and radish to one side and put the rest of the vegetables into a mixing bowl with the chopped herb.

In a small container with a sealable lid (or jam jar), make the dressing from the mead reduction and the rapeseed (canola) oil and shake well. Add half of this dressing to the salad in the bowl and toss until coated.

To serve, arrange the dressed salad on 2 plates or bowls, around the edges divide the cheese quenelles, beetroot, radish and asparagus between them. Flake the salmon into bite-sized pieces and sit this on top of the salad and top with a final drizzle of the dressing over the salmon. Garnish with the chervil or sweet cicely.

 Balance Add 75g (2½oz) cold sliced new potatoes coated in the remaining dressing and season to taste.

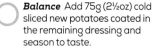 **Build** Add the potatoes as in Balance, plus enjoy with a couple of rye crackers or some thinly sliced rye bread.

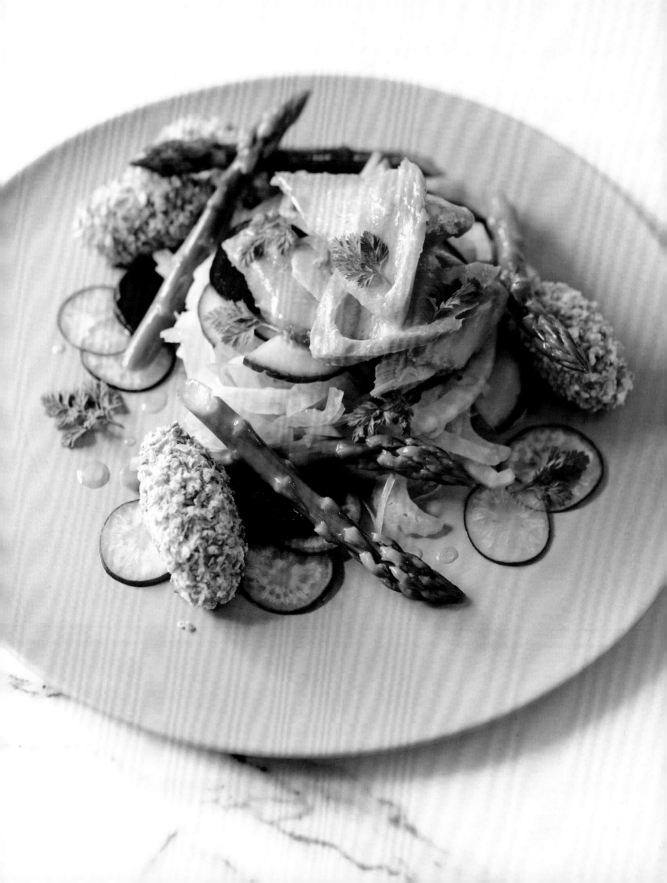

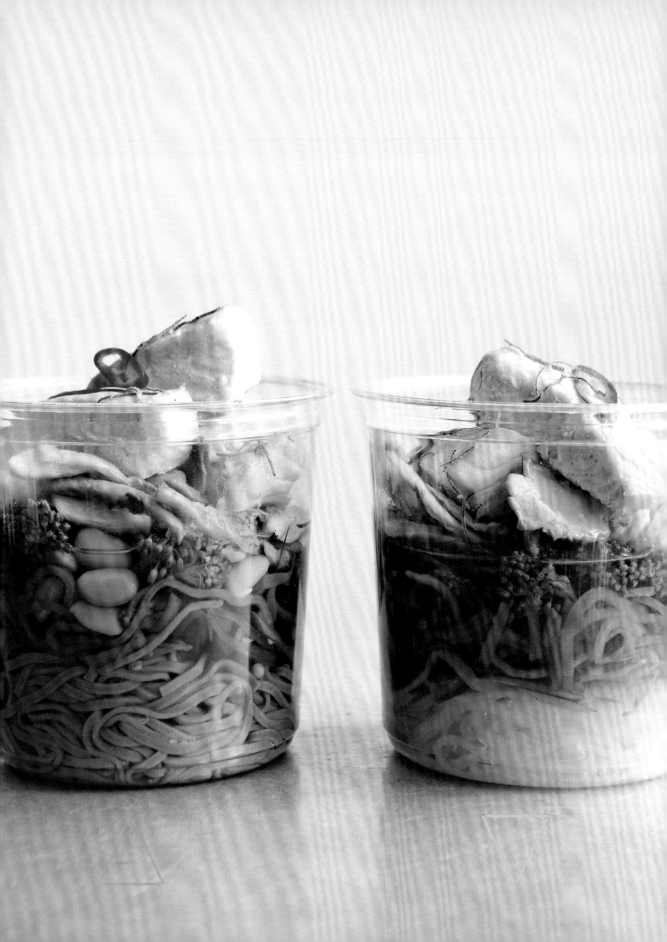

Salmon with oyster mushrooms and buckwheat noodles

This Asian-inspired salmon dish is light and authentic. Make the broth in advance for a speedy, nutritious and umami-laden midweek dinner.

Health The oyster mushrooms provide a good amount of your daily intake of niacin to help counter any digestive problems or fatigue.

Sport The salmon's omega-3 fatty acids can help improve the omega-3:omega-6 ratio, reducing inflammation and perhaps even injuries.

SERVES 2

2 skinless salmon fillets (about 140g/5oz each)
1 carrot
60g (2¼oz) sugar snap peas
100g (3½oz) tenderstem broccoli
3 spring onions (scallions), sliced
80g (3¼oz) oyster mushrooms
1 tsp vegetable oil
sea salt and freshly ground black pepper
100g (3½oz) buckwheat noodles
4 sage leaves, finely sliced to garnish
1 red chilli, sliced to garnish

FOR THE BROTH:

3 tsp kuzu
5g organic vegetable bouillon (½ cube or 1½ tsp powder)
500ml (2 cups) water
1 tsp fish sauce
2 tsp tamari (or soy sauce)
1 tbsp mirin
1 tsp chopped root ginger
1 star anise
1 clove garlic, chopped
1 tsp ground dried kombu
1 red chilli, deseeded and chopped

Preheat the oven to 180°C/350°F/gas mark 4, and line a baking tray (cookie sheet) with baking parchment.

Make the broth by mixing the kuzu and the bouillon in some of the water. Add this and the rest of the ingredients to a pan and bring to the boil. Remove from the heat and allow the flavours to infuse for 20 minutes. Then, strain through a fine sieve (strainer) and return to the pan.

Next, place the salmon fillets onto the prepared baking tray (cookie sheet) and cook in a preheated oven for 8–10 minutes until done.

Meanwhile, finely slice the carrot into thin batons (or use a mandolin). Cut the sugar snaps in half on an angle and trim the stalks of the tenderstem broccoli, if necessary.

Bring the broth back to the boil and add the carrots, boil for 3 minutes then add the broccoli. Boil for a further 3 minutes then add the spring onions and the sugar snaps. Turn off the heat and leave to rest.

Pull any large mushrooms apart into smaller pieces and place in a hot frying pan over a high heat with the oil and cook for 2–2½ minutes until browned a little and softened. Season with salt, to taste.

Cook the noodles in a pan of boiling water until soft. Drain through a sieve (strainer) and serve.

To serve, divide the noodles between 2 bowls along with half of the vegetables and the broth. Place half of the mushrooms and a piece of salmon on top of each and garnish with the sage and chilli.

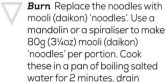

Burn Replace the noodles with mooli (daikon) 'noodles'. Use a mandolin or a spiraliser to make 80g (3¼oz) mooli (daikon) 'noodles' per portion. Cook these in a pan of boiling salted water for 2 minutes, drain and serve.

Build Include 70g (2½oz) edamame per portion; add these to the broth when you add the broccoli.

Halloumi, salsa verde and pasta salad

This salad has something for everyone! Halloumi, cherry tomatoes, rocket (arugula) and olives combine to make a stunning salad dish for lunch that can easily be thrown together for a BBQ with family and friends.

Health The fennel seeds promote excellent digestive function and reduce bloating.

Sport Halloumi is a great source of vegetarian protein to help support muscle protein synthesis.

SERVES 2

100g (3½oz) wholewheat penne pasta

small bunch flat-leaf parsley

2 anchovies, drained

2 tsp capers, drained

½ tsp white wine vinegar

2 tsp extra virgin olive oil

80g (3¼oz) cherry tomatoes, quartered

25g (¼ cup) pitted black olives, chopped

15g (½oz) Parmesan, shaved with a vegetable peeler

½ tsp fennel seeds

finely grated zest of ½ lemon

25g (1oz) rocket (arugula)

200g (7oz) low-fat halloumi

Cook the pasta in a large pan of boiling water until cooked to your liking. Drain, cool under cold running water and set aside.

Meanwhile, in a beaker using a hand-held blender, blitz the parsley, anchovies, capers, vinegar and olive oil to form a rough paste – this is the salsa verde.

In a large bowl, mix the tomatoes, olives, half of the Parmesan shavings, the fennel seeds, lemon zest and rocket (arugula) together. Add the pasta and half of the salsa verde and gently fold until all is coated.

Slice the block of halloumi into 12 pieces and cook in a hot non-stick frying pan (skillet) over a high heat on each side until golden brown.

Divide the pasta salad between 2 bowls and top each with half of the halloumi and the rest of the Parmesan then share out the remaining salsa verde.

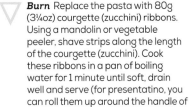

Burn Replace the pasta with 80g (3¼oz) courgette (zucchini) ribbons. Using a mandolin or vegetable peeler, shave strips along the length of the courgette (zucchini). Cook these ribbons in a pan of boiling water for 1 minute until soft, drain well and serve (for presentatino, you can roll them up around the handle of a wooden spoon if desired).

Build Increase the portion size of the pasta to 80g (¼oz) per portion.

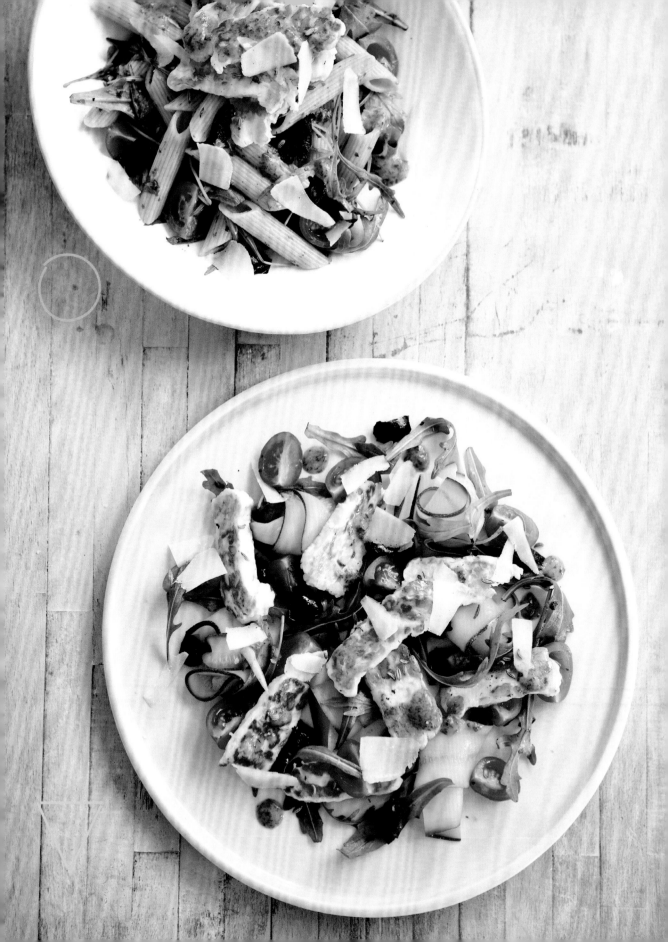

Kimchi silken stew

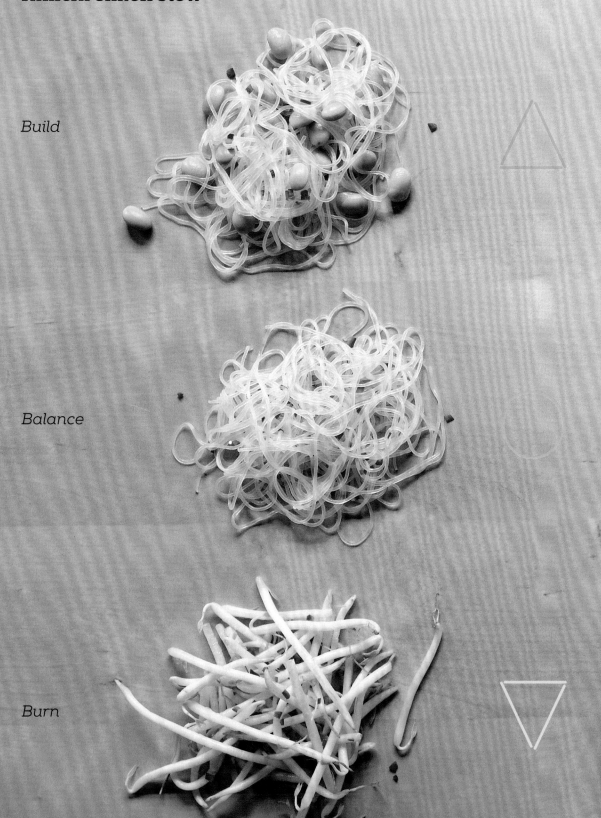

Build

Balance

Burn

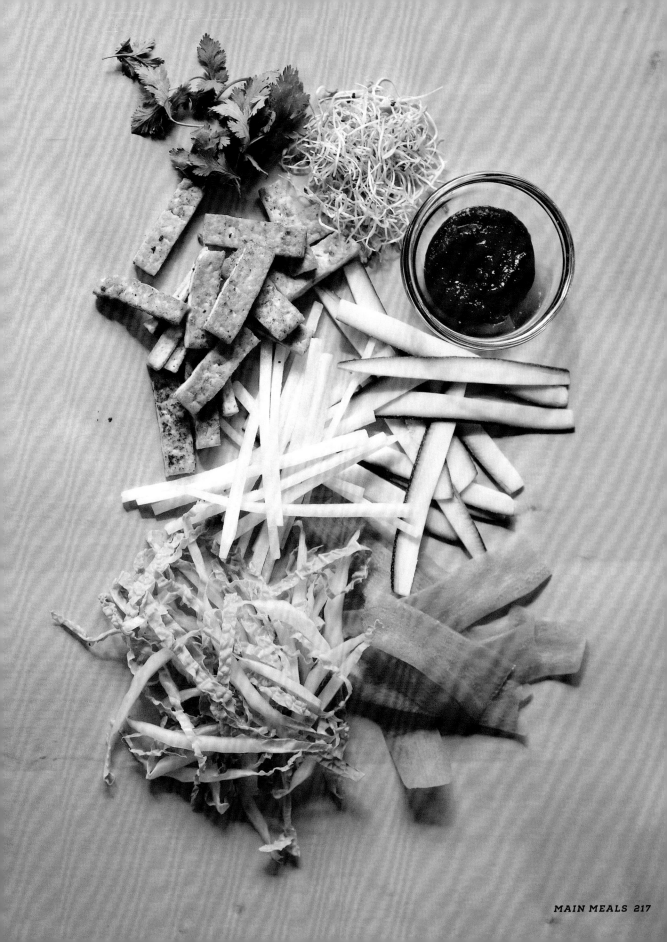

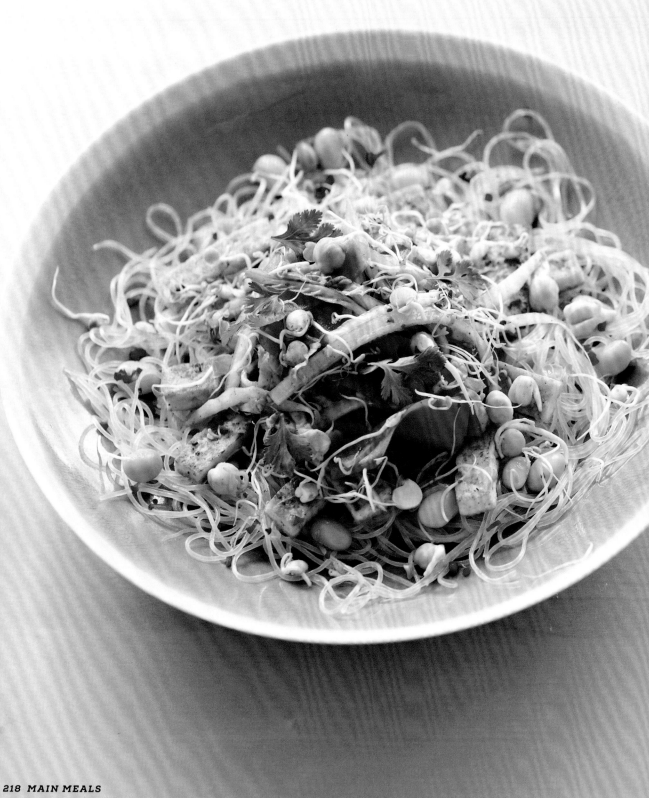

Kimchi silken stew

Transport yourself to Asia with this fresh and aromatic dish that will tantalise your taste buds, Korean-style.

Top tip If you're not a fan of tofu, toss some sliced chicken breast in a little Korean paste and fry in a pan before adding to the stew at the end.

Health The silken tofu in this dish provides a great source of vegan protein for those who don't eat meat.

SERVES 2

FOR THE PICKLING LIQUOR:

550ml (scant 2½ cups) Kimchi pickle liquor

200ml (scant 1 cup) white wine vinegar

20g (3 tsp) agave syrup

2g (pinch) coriander (cilantro), chopped

½ tsp Korean hot pepper paste

150ml (⅔ cup) water

FOR THE STEW:

70g (2½oz) sweet heart cabbage, shredded

1 carrot, thinly sliced

1 small courgette (zucchini), thinly sliced

90g (3¼oz) mooli (daikon), thinly sliced

80g (3¼oz) silken tofu

1 tbsp vegetable oil

½ tsp Korean hot pepper paste

5g (⅛oz) organic vegetable bouillon (½ cube or 1½ tsp powder)

300ml (1¼ cups) water

1 tsp tamari

2 tbsp kuzu

1 tsp roasted garlic paste (see page 106)

sea salt and freshly ground black pepper

300g (10½oz) cooked rice noodles

Mix together all the pickling liquor ingredients in a large bowl and add the cabbage, carrot, courgette (zucchini) and mooli (daikon). Leave for 1 hour, then drain.

Meanwhile, bring a large pan of salted water to the boil then carefully add the tofu and simmer for 4 minutes until slightly firm and puffed up. Using a slotted spoon, transfer the tofu into a bowl and set aside.

Heat the oil in a large heavy pan, add the Korean paste and cook for 2 minutes. Add the vegetable bouillon and water then bring to the boil. Reduce the heat and simmer for 30 minutes then add the tofu, pickled vegetables, tamari, kuzu, roasted garlic paste and season to taste, using tamari or soy sauce.

To serve, divide the cooked rice noodles between 2 bowls and ladle the stew on top.

Burn Substitute 150g (1½ cups) beansprouts per portion for the rice noodles.

 Build Add 30g (1oz) edamame per portion to the rice noodles.

Pumpkin cannelloni with roasted vegetables

With its classical Italian heritage, this vegetarian dish stands on its own without the need for meat to enhance the flavour. It's served with a vibrant spinach and basil sauce for extra wow factor.

Top tip If you're serving these to guests, then make the cannelloni in advance and store in a sealed container; they take just a few minutes to reheat in the microwave or oven.

Sport This dish provides a great intake of calcium to help maintain bone health and density – an important aspect for those sportspeople who compete in non-weight-bearing activities.

SERVES 2

FOR THE CANNELLONI:

130g (4½oz) butternut squash or pumpkin, diced

160g (¾ cup) low-fat cream cheese

¼ tsp lemon thyme leaves

sea salt and freshly ground black pepper

4 fresh egg lasagne sheets

FOR THE ROASTED VEGETABLES:

½ small onion, diced

100g (3½oz) baby corn, sliced

180g (6½oz) cherry or baby plum tomatoes

50g (½ cup) black olives, pitted

1 tsp vegetable oil

FOR THE SAUCE:

120ml (½ cup) water

1½ tsp cornflour (cornstarch)

2.5g organic vegetable bouillon (¼ cube or ¾ tsp powder)

150g (5½oz) spinach

15g (generous ⅓ cup) basil

sea salt

In a large pan with several litres (quarts) of water add the diced squash and bring to the boil. Cook until soft but not falling apart. Drain through a sieve (strainer) and return to the pan. Then, add the cream cheese, lemon thyme and seasoning to taste.

Preheat the oven to 220°C/425°F/gas mark 7, and you'll need a baking tray (cookie sheet).

Preheat an electric steamer or use a nest steamer over a pan of boiling water. Place a sheet of the lasagne into the steamer and cook for 2 minutes until softened slightly. Remove from the steamer and place onto a chopping (cutting) board. Spoon one-quarter of the squash and cheese mixture evenly along the shortest edge (have the shortest edge nearest you so it's easy to roll away to make the cannelloni). Roll the lasagne to create a tube with the mixture inside, overlapping the end by 2.5–3cm (1–1¼in) and trimming off any excess. Repeat this with the other lasagne sheets.

Meanwhile, put the onion, baby corn, tomatoes and olives on a baking tray (cookie sheet), drizzle with the oil and roast in a preheated oven for 8–10 minutes. Place the now-assembled four cannelloni back into the steamer and steam for 6–8 minutes.

Meanwhile, in a cup mix a little of the water with the cornflour (cornstarch) to form a paste then stir in the rest of the water. Place this along with the vegetable bouillon into a large pan with a lid and bring to the boil. While it's boiling add the spinach and the basil and stir. Put the lid on and bring back to the boil to wilt the spinach. Transfer the contents of the pan to a jug blender and blitz until smooth (or, if you prefer, use a beaker and hand-held blender). Then, return the smooth sauce to the pan and add a little salt to taste, then reheat and serve. To plate up, place 2 cannelloni and half of the roasted vegetables onto each plate, then pour over the hot sauce and serve immediately.

 Burn Make the filling as per the recipe but use aubergines (eggplants) to contain the filling instead of lasagne. Roast 4 baby white aubergines (eggplants) for 20 minutes at 170°C/344°F/gas mark 3 and then cut the tops off, hollow them out, stuff them with the mix then put them back in the oven for 15–20 minutes until piping hot.

 Build Serve with 2 slices of granary garlic bread for those extra carbs (but go easy on the butter). To make the garlic bread, preheat the oven to 220°C/425°F/gas mark 7. Slice a granary baguette at an angle (about 2cm/¾in thick) to make the required quantity. Mix 1 tsp of spreadable light butter with either ¼ teaspoon of roasted garlic paste (see page 106) or ¼ clove of finely chopped garlic and add a pinch of chopped parsley per portion. Spread evenly over each slice and bake on a tray in a preheated oven for 5–6 minutes.

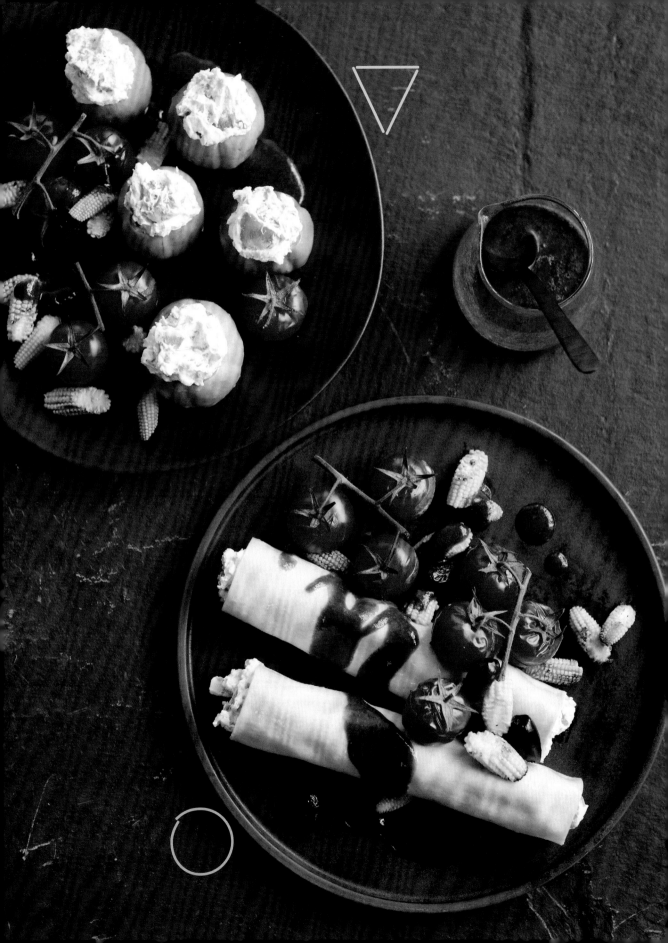

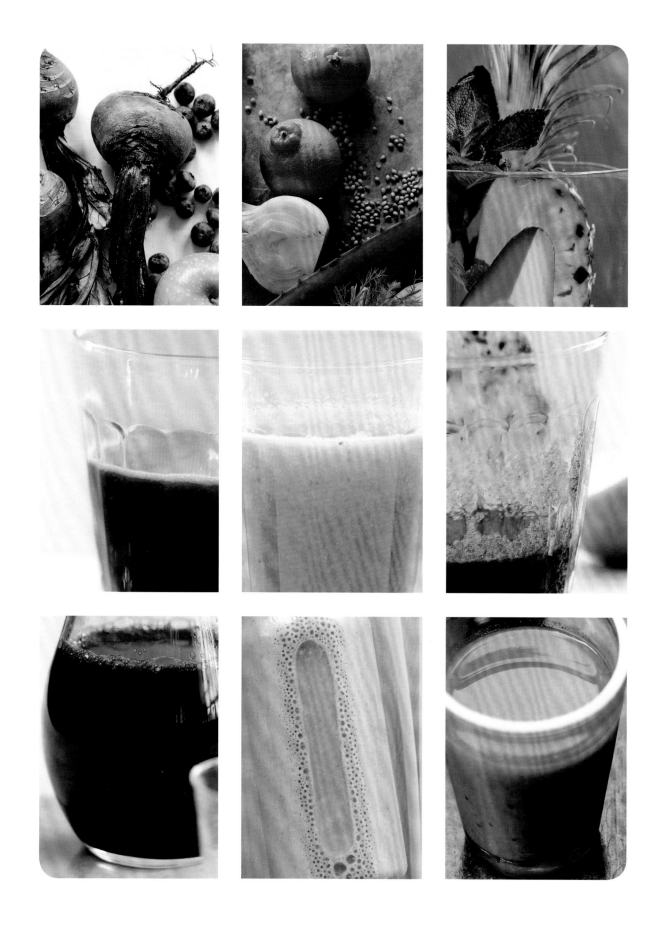

JUICES, SHAKES & SMOOTHIES

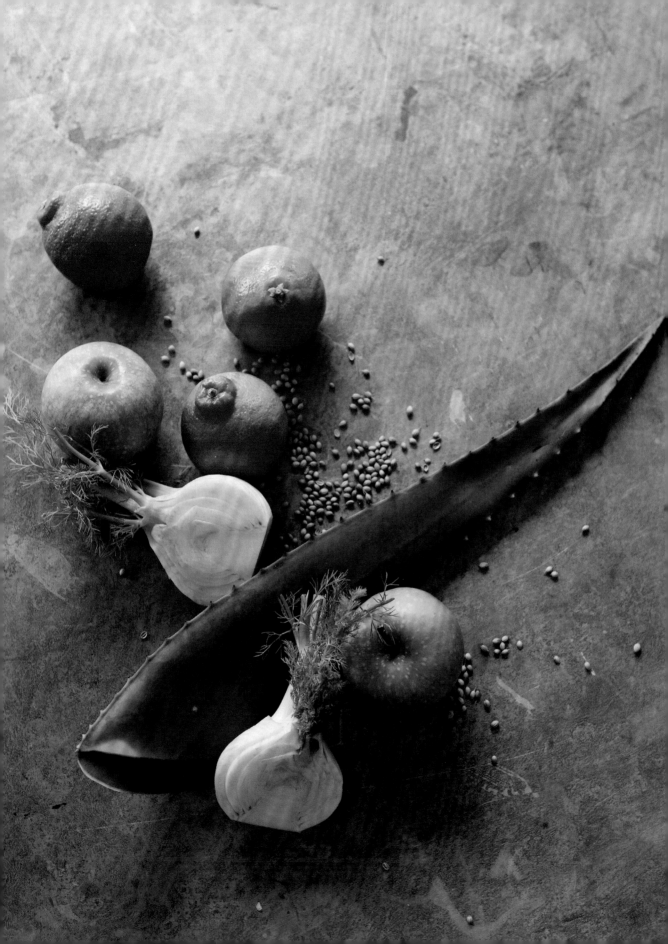

Clean

The mild aniseed flavour from the fennel and the sweetness of the apple and mandarin create a lovely clean and refreshing taste. The coriander seeds offset any bitterness and make this cleansing cocktail sing!

Health Many people take aloe vera to help with digestion but it is also great for supporting immunity, cleansing and for clear and healthy-looking skin.

Top tip Feel free to switch the coriander seeds for a handful of uplifting mint if the mood takes you!

SERVES 2

1 bulb fennel

2 mandarin

2 Granny Smith apples, cored

25ml (5 tsp) aloe vera juice

10 coriander seeds, crushed

Simply put all the ingredients through a juicer. This juice is best drunk straightaway but keeps for 24 hours in the fridge.

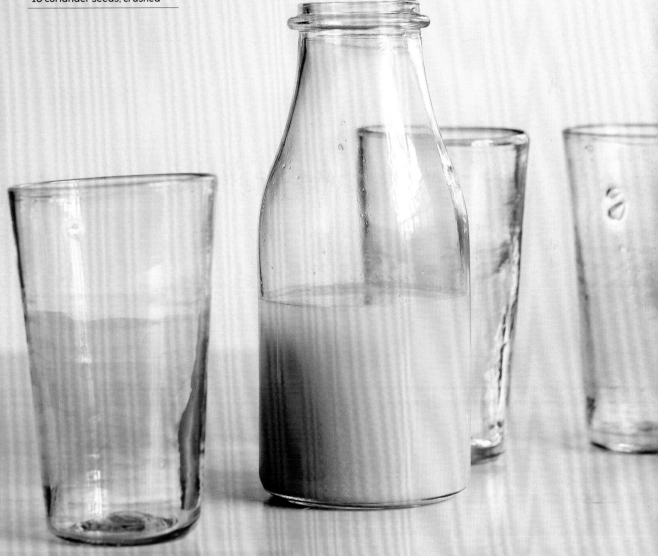

Proconut – Raw cacao

The electrolytes in coconut water make it one of the best ways of rehydrating and in this shake it is combined with banana and cocoa – what's not to like?

Health The theobromine component of raw cacao is a non-addictive stimulant; some research has shown it can treat depression.

Sport All proconut shakes contain at least 25g (1oz) protein so are perfect to maximise protein synthesis after training.

SERVES 2

200ml (scant 1 cup) coconut water

150ml (⅔ cup) cashew milk

1 banana, puréed

14g (2½ tbsp) raw cacao powder

6g (1 tbsp) cocoa powder

60g (2¼oz) unflavoured whey protein

Simply put all the ingredients into a jug blender and whizz until really smooth. This shake is best drunk straightaway but keeps for 24 hours in the fridge.

Proconut – Pina colada

This nutritious and super-hydrating coconut-water-based shake captures all the flavours of a beachside cocktail but with nothing but goodness!

Health Pineapple is an excellent source of manganese – an essential factor in energy production and antioxidant defence.

Sport Proconut drinks are all higher in calories than other juices so use them when you need to up your calorie intake.

SERVES 2

150ml (⅔ cup) coconut milk

120ml (½ cup) coconut water

1 small banana, puréed

100ml (scant ½ cup) pineapple juice

60g (2¼oz) unflavoured whey protein

Simply put all the ingredients into a jug blender and whizz until really smooth. This shake is best drunk straightaway but keeps for 24 hours in the fridge.

Proconut – Alkaline greens

This coconut-based drink is quick and easy to make and tastes amazing. This shake delivers protein, iron, dietary fibre and electrolytes for rehydration.

Health Spirulina (a natural 'algae' powder) is incredibly high in essential amino acids, which will keep your muscles healthy.

Sport With its combination of protein and rehydrating electrolytes, this drink does the job of meeting your body's post-training needs.

SERVES 2

100ml (scant ½ cup) coconut milk

110ml (scant ½ cup) coconut water

1 small banana

½ apple

1 tbsp lemon juice

½ tsp grated root ginger

2 tsp spirulina

35g (1¼oz) lychee

60g (2¼oz) unflavoured whey protein

40g (1½oz) spinach

Simply put all the ingredients into a jug blender and whizz until really smooth. This shake is best drunk straightaway but keeps for 24 hours in the fridge.

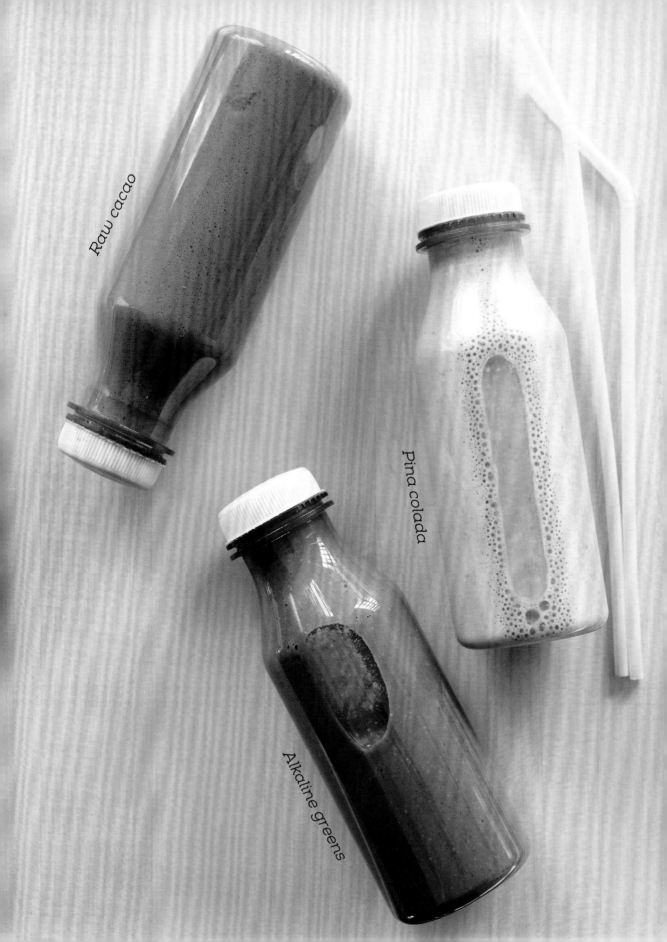

Raw cacao

Pina colada

Alkaline greens

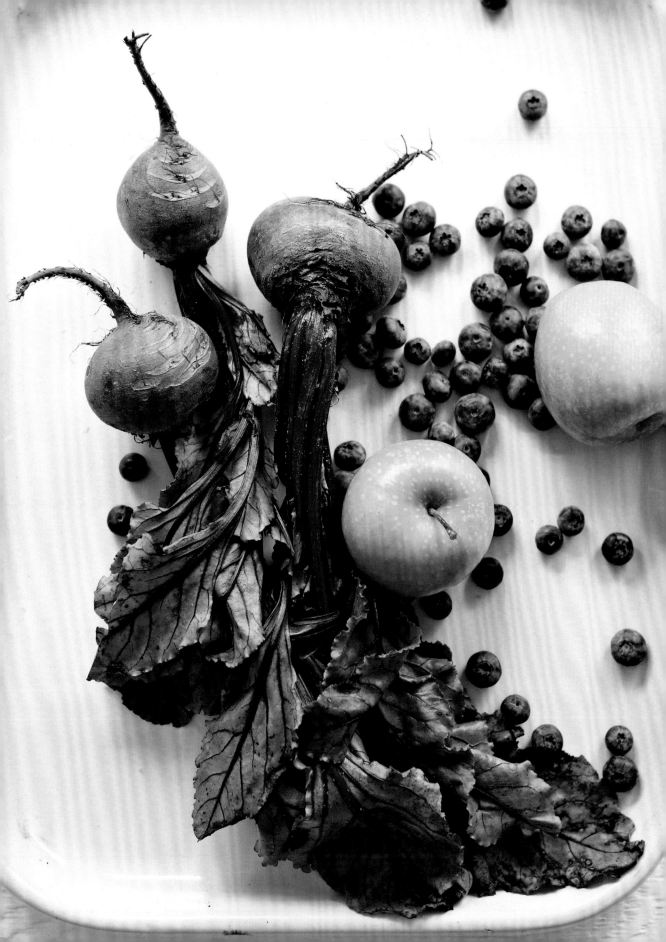

Up beet

Start your day with this refreshing and energising beetroot combo. The beetroot gives a deliciously earthy note, which is complemented by the sweetness of the apple. And when combined with the blueberries, you get the most stunning colour as well as a bunch of vitamins, antioxidants and dietary fibre.

Health Beetroot is so good for you: it is high in potassium and fibre and is a great source of vitamin C.

Sport Chemicals in the beetroot help with the uptake of oxygen in the body, so will fire you up for your next training session.

SERVES 2

300g (10½oz) raw beetroot

300g (2 cups) blueberries (use blackcurrants when in season)

3 Granny Smith apples, cored

Simply put all the ingredients through a juicer. This juice is best drunk straightaway but keeps for up to 3 days in the fridge.

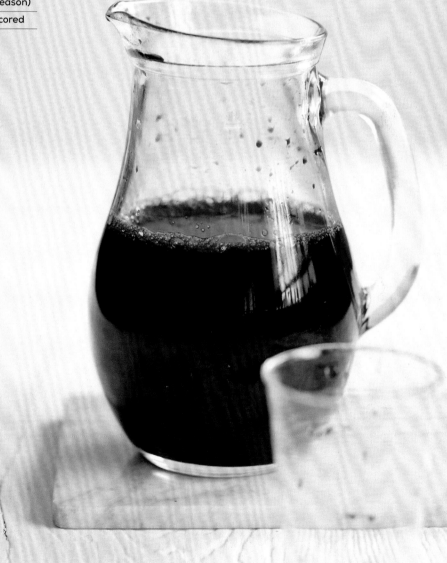

Very berry

The deep-coloured berries used in this smoothie mean that not only does it taste great but it's packed full of antioxidants, especially from using black grapes, which has the best nutrition profile of all grapes.

Health Studies have shown that the low GI value of grapes, when consumed regularly, results in better blood sugar balance and better insulin regulation.

Sport The yogurt in the smoothie gives you a source of protein and fat. If you need to cut down on fat, use a low-fat Greek yogurt instead.

▽
SERVES 2

150g (5oz) black grapes

75g (½ cup) blueberries

75g (½ cup) blackberries

50g (¼ cup) Greek yogurt

100ml (scant ½ cup) apple juice

Simply put all the ingredients into a jug blender and whizz until really smooth. This smoothie is best drunk straightaway but keeps for 24 hours in the fridge.

Kickstart

This citrus-fruit-based juice is packed full of beta-carotene and immunity-boosting vitamin C – the perfect antidote if you feel a cold coming on.

Health The bitter nature of this juice also means that it digests to become very alkaline, which is perfect for balancing out the typically acidic Western diet.

Sport Red chilli peppers reduce blood cholesterol and triglyceride (another fat in your blood) levels, helping to keep your cardiovascular system in tip-top shape.

▽
SERVES 2

2 blood oranges

420g (15oz) carrots, peeled and topped

¼ pomello

1.5cm (⅝in) cube root ginger

½ small red chilli

Simply put all the ingredients into a jug blender and whizz until really smooth. This smoothie is best drunk straightaway but keeps for 24 hours in the fridge.

Reset

Probably the freshest-tasting of all of our juices or smoothies, this vitamin-packed booster is ideal for helping to balance a lower-calorie diet.

Health Containing more vitamin C than an orange, kiwi fruits are packed with all sorts of beneficial phytonutrients.

Sport Spirulina is a great vegan source of protein – add more if you like the taste to supercharge your smoothie with protein.

SERVES 2

- 2 Granny Smith apples, cored
- 2 kiwi fruits, peeled
- 160g (5¾oz) cucumber
- juice of 1 lime
- 4g (⅛oz) mint leaves
- 2 tsp spirulina
- 200ml (scant 1 cup) apple juice

Simply put all the ingredients into a jug blender and whizz until really smooth. This smoothie is best drunk straightaway but keeps for 24 hours in the fridge.

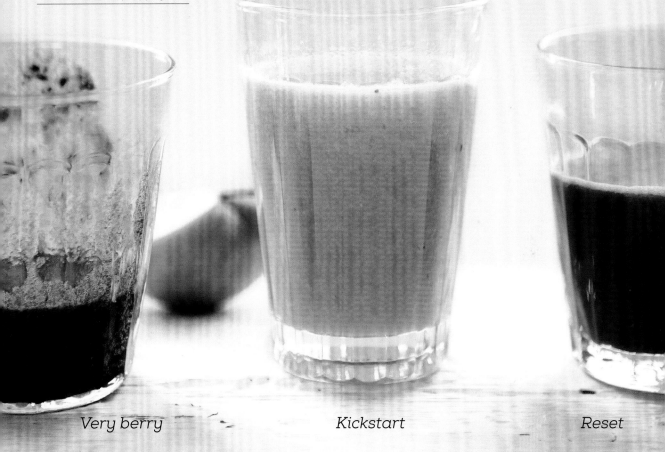

Very berry   *Kickstart*   *Reset*

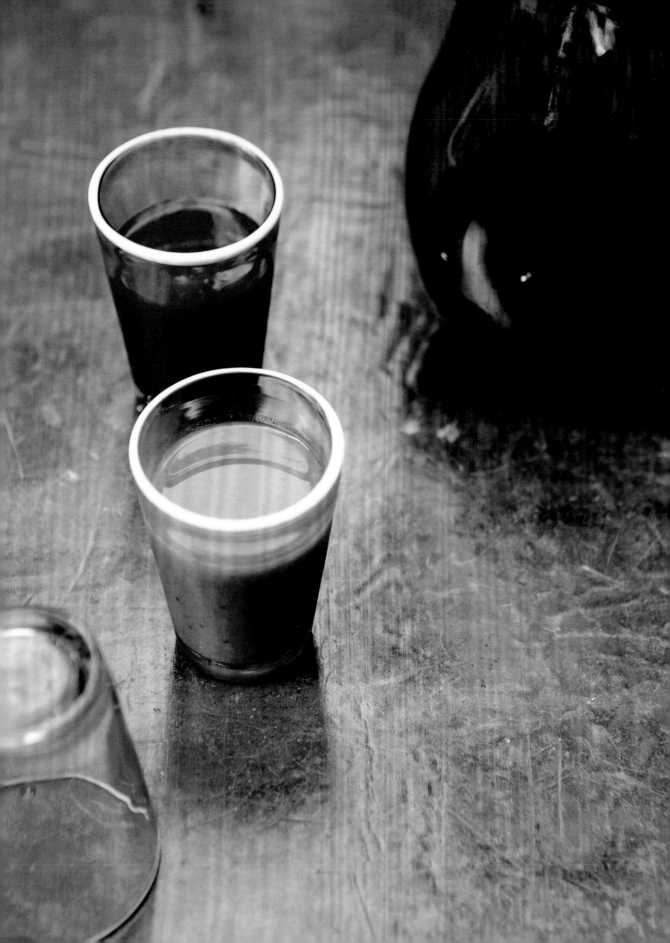

Heartbeet

This vibrant juice is good for your heart. Red and purple vegetables and fruit contain antioxidant chemicals such as anthocyanins and lycopene that can help fight heart disease.

Top tip Take your smoothie with you to work in a thermos flask for a mid-morning or afternoon snack. Just give it a good shake first before drinking.

Sport Dietary nitrates reduce the 'energy cost of exercise', allowing a higher power output for the same oxygen consumption – you get more energy and better performance when working out.

SERVES 2

150g (5½oz) beetroot, half peeled

360g (12½oz) pears

120g (4½oz) apricots or plums (whatever's in season), destoned

35 pomegranate seeds

Simply put all the ingredients through a juicer. This juice is best drunk straightaway but keeps for 24 hours in the fridge.

Glow

Glow is an edible tonic to nourish your skin and hair from the inside out. Tap into the power of cucumber – they are 96 per cent water so make the perfect juicing veggie. The ginger has antiseptic properties and can help to keep skin clear and blemish free. Give it a glow!

Health Apples are loaded with beta carotene and apple peel is particularly rich in polyphenols. Both of these offer antioxidant and anti-inflammatory protection to slow down the aging of skin.

Sport This juice's levels of vitamin K help it to boost bone density and benefit your general bone health, which is especially important for those doing repetitive high-impact sports, such as triathlon and distance running.

SERVES 2

100g (3½oz) celery, stalks cut in half

3 Granny Smith apples, cored

100g (3½oz) cucumber

1 lemon, peeled

a thumb-sized piece of root ginger, peeled

Simply put all the ingredients through a juicer. This juice is best drunk straightaway but keeps for 24 hours in the fridge.

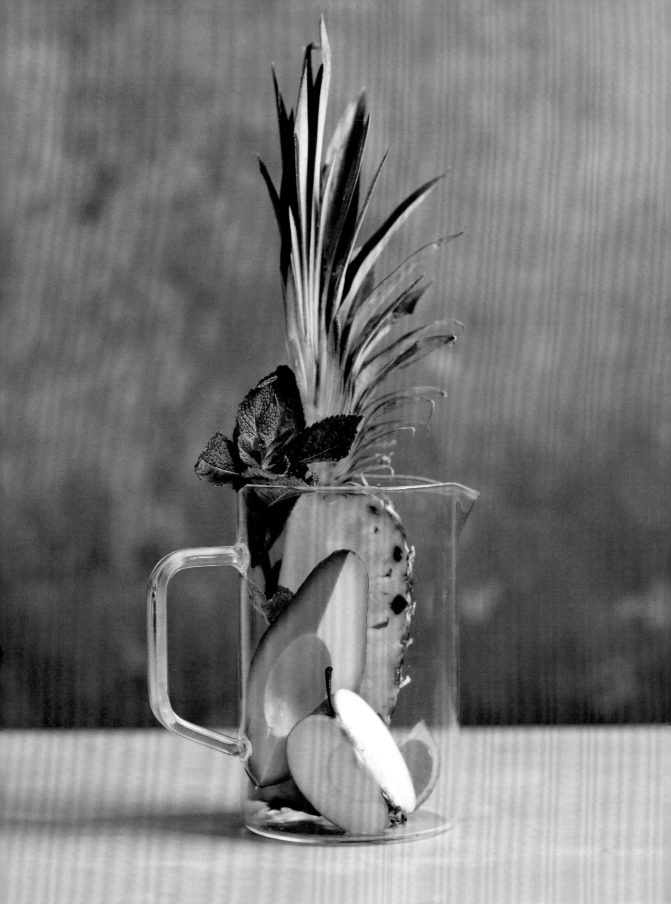

Radiance

Radiate from within with this colourful juice that's perfect for breakfast. The avocado in this smoothie makes it dreamily creamy and smooth but also adds some much-needed healthy fats. Pineapple offers plenty of tropical flavour while the mint freshens it up.

Health As well as delivering plant-based nutrients, avocados offer the right amount and combination of dietary fats, including the monounsaturated fatty acid oleic acid.

Top tip If the smoothie is too thick for you, add a little cold water to thin it out.

SERVES 2

1 avocado

¼ pineapple

4 mint leaves

juice of ½ lime

2 Granny Smith apples, cored

Simply put all the ingredients into a jug blender and whizz until really smooth. This smoothie is best drunk straightaway but keeps for 24 hours in the fridge.

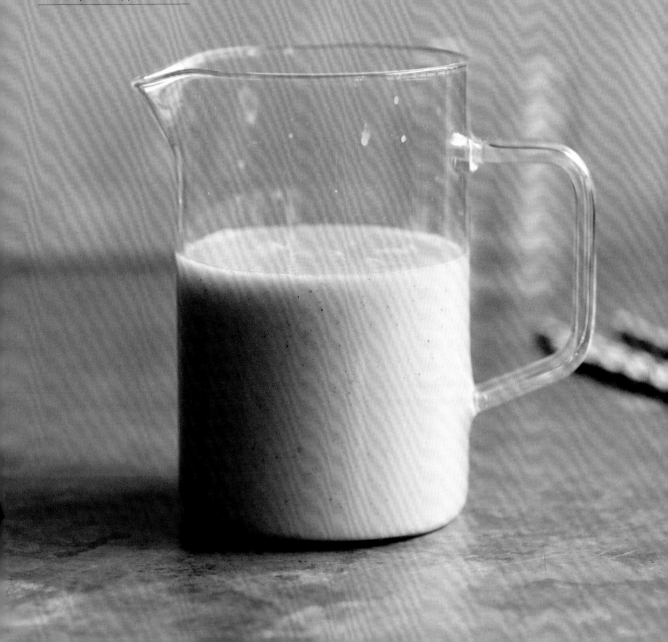

Vitality

The mixing of celery and grapefruit may sound unusual but both share matching points of their flavour profiles to provide a great-tasting combination for optimal health and vitality.

Health Phytonutrients called limonoids in grapefruit may prevent cancer. They promote the formation of a detoxifying enzyme, which helps the body excrete toxic compounds better.

Sport As well as supporting immunity, vitamin C promotes the growth and repair of tissues in all parts of your body. So, if you're training hard, be sure to top up the vitamin C levels.

SERVES 2

| 420g (15oz) carrots, peeled and topped |
| 2 sticks celery |
| 1 grapefruit |

Simply put all the ingredients through a juicer. This juice is best drunk straightaway but keeps for 24 hours in the fridge. Use the pulp to make Carrot and caraway crackers, see page 106.

Energiser

Drink this juice like a summer punch – pour into a tall glass over ice, sit back and relax, while the juice works wonders for your health and energy levels.

Health Nectarines contain a substance called lutein, which helps keep your eyes and skin healthy. But it's also an important antioxidant, helping to destroy harmful free radicals in your body.

Sport Low potassium can cause muscle cramping and cardiovascular issues so it's good to know that passionfruit supplies a great potassium-laden punch. So, no more cramps during workouts!

SERVES 2

| 300g (2 cups) strawberries |
| 400g (14oz) tomatoes |
| 2 passionfruit |
| 4 nectarines |

Simply put all the ingredients through a juicer. This juice is best drunk straightaway but keeps for 24 hours in the fridge.

Boost

One for 'The King' perhaps, who had a penchant for banana and peanut butter sandwiches. This sweet and nutty shake is designed for cramming in extra calories for post-workout recovery or muscle growth. We're sure Elvis would approve.

Health In addition to their monounsaturated fat content, peanuts supply many other heart-healthy nutrients – vitamin E, niacin, folate, protein and manganese.

Top tip Prepare this shake before training, pop in a bottle or flask and have it handy for a super-quick recovery boost. Add a scoop of flavoured or unflavoured whey to up the protein levels if you like.

SERVES 2

| 2 bananas |
| 50g (⅓ cup) unsalted peanuts |
| ¼ tsp ground nutmeg |
| 2 tsp honey |
| 350ml (1½ cups) skimmed milk |

Simply put all the ingredients into a jug blender and whizz until really smooth. This shake is best drunk straightaway but keeps for 24 hours in the fridge.

Index

Acknowledgements

The are quite a number of people that I would like to thank for giving me the opportunity to create this book, as well as bringing it to life and making it real. Firstly, my parents for their continued support and my mum for being such a bad cook that it really spurred me on in my younger years to be more creative in the kitchen!

Tracey Woodward is the best fairy godmother anyone could have! The doors you have opened and the help you have given me along the years is something that I will be forever grateful for.

I'd like to thank all my team at Soulmatefood, especially Miles Ridley for your innovation and cheese and wine, Tom for validation and knowledge plus Tina and Duncan for holding everything together!

Thanks to Mark Ellison for some amazing opportunities and all the guys at Virgin for building such a strong partnership.

Last but not least, I would like to thank Jacqui, Fritha, Nikki, Lawrence, Cynthia and Yuki for being so patient, supportive and an amazing bunch to work with.